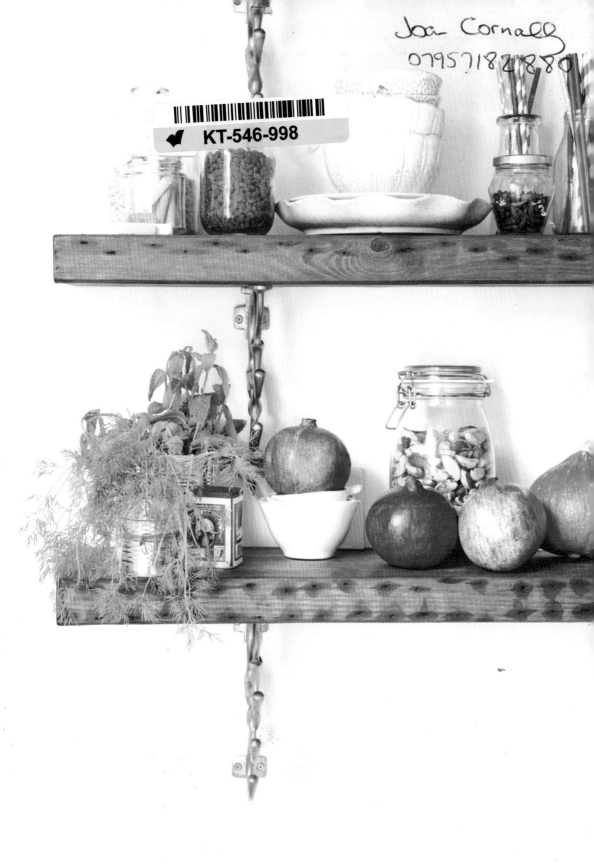

Joa Cornall
07957182880

Deliciously
Ella

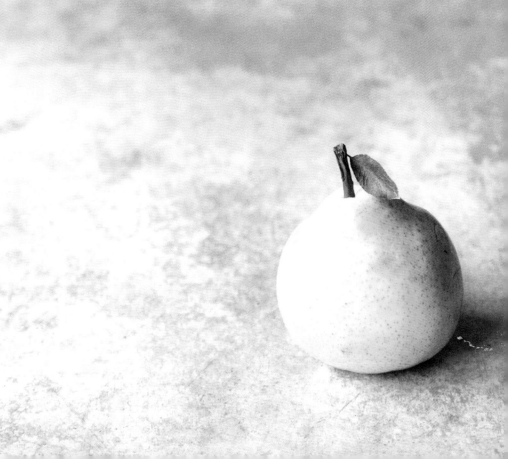

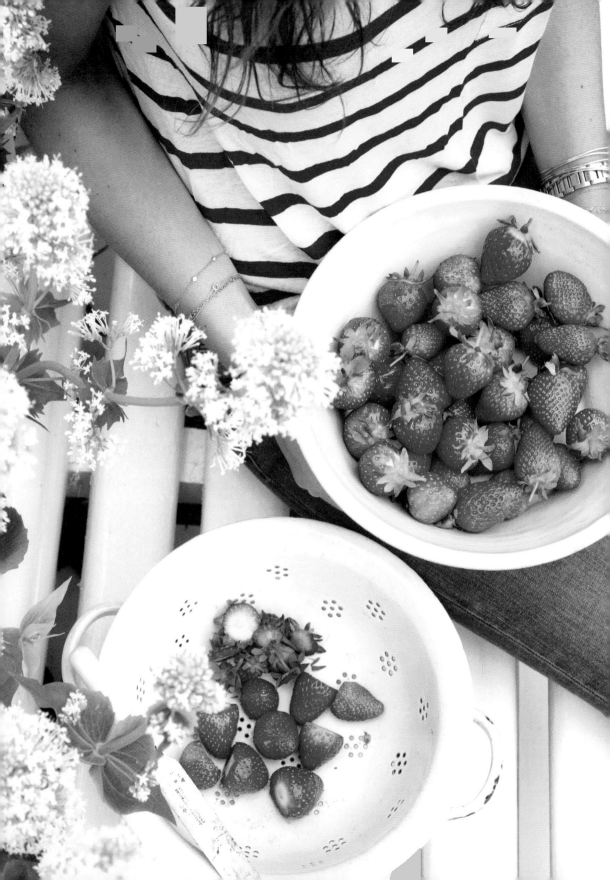

Deliciously Ella

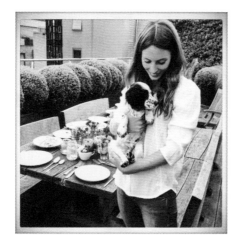

Awesome
ingredients and
incredible food
that you and
your body
will love

Ella Woodward

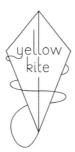

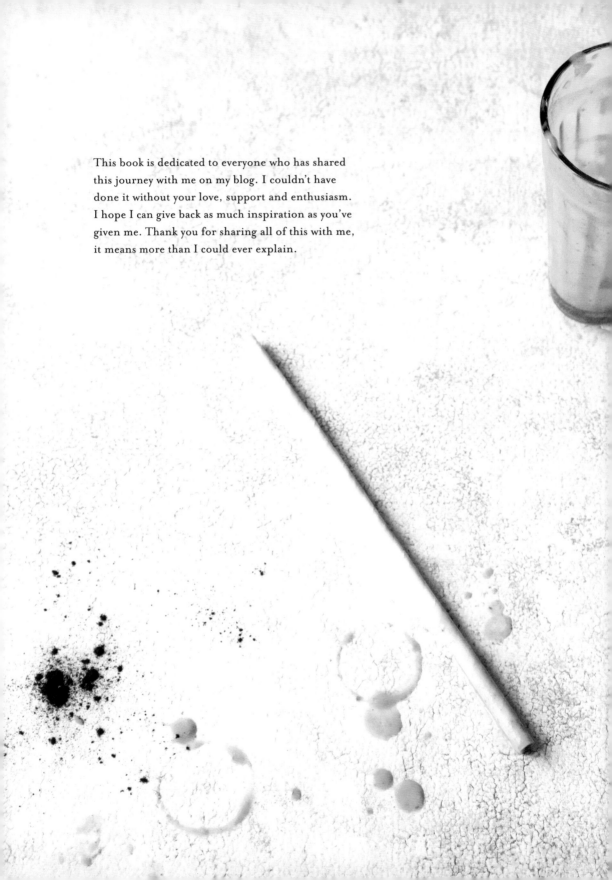

This book is dedicated to everyone who has shared
this journey with me on my blog. I couldn't have
done it without your love, support and enthusiasm.
I hope I can give back as much inspiration as you've
given me. Thank you for sharing all of this with me,
it means more than I could ever explain.

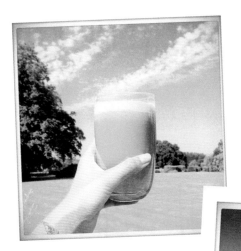

CONTENTS

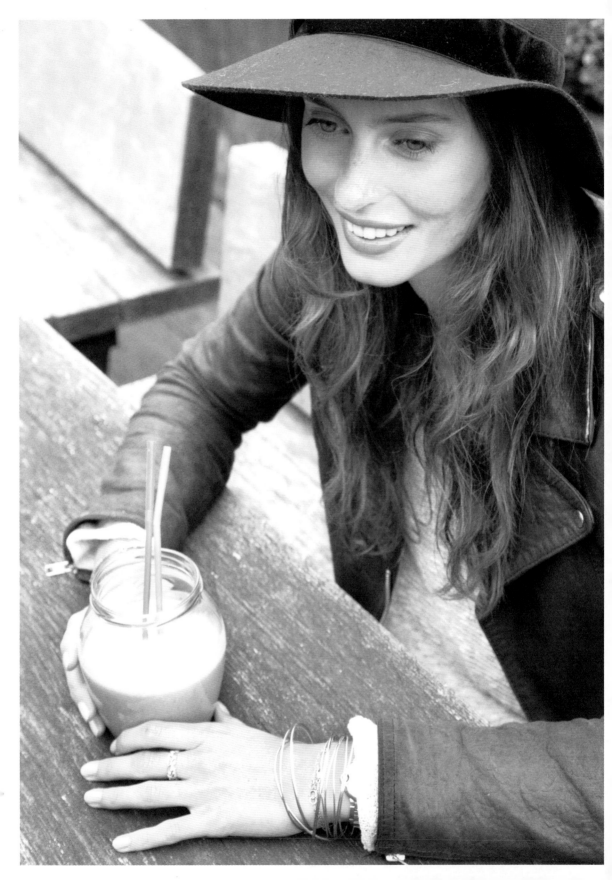

MY STORY

Until just over four years ago I was a sugar monster, and I mean a total addict. I'd always had a serious sweet tooth and as a child my favourite foods were sprinkle sandwiches and what we liked to call chocolate mess. Chocolate mess was pretty amazing, and just as sticky as it sounds. To make it my sisters and I would raid our kitchen cupboards for anything sweet and throw together whatever we could find into a bowl – usually a mix of milk chocolate, marshmallows, gummy sweets, caramel, golden syrup and Rice Krispies – which we'd melt in a saucepan until it formed a gooey pile of chocolate deliciousness. The three of us would then sit with our teaspoons and demolish the whole bowl! My love of sugar grew from there, peaking during my first year of university in St Andrews when my friends and I basically lived off a delicious mixture of Ben & Jerry's Cookie Dough ice cream, mountains of chocolate (preferably filled with gooey caramel) and lots of fizzy pick 'n' mix. We were all totally hooked on sugar-laden convenience foods, and nutrition was low on the priority list!

It seems crazy that my diet has transformed so dramatically in such a relatively short amount of time, and I'm sure that as you flip through this book you'll have a hard time believing that I used to eat this way. It will probably seem even crazier still when I tell you that I actually didn't like any fruits or vegetables, but I promise you I really didn't! Other than bananas and corn on the cob I steered clear of anything fruit or veg related.

Things all changed really quickly though, and very unexpectedly. In the summer of 2011, just after I'd finished my second year of university, I was diagnosed with a relatively rare illness called Postural Tachycardia Syndrome, or POTS. It's a very strange illness and even now my closest family and friends can't quite get their heads around it. The syndrome effectively breaks down your autonomic nervous system: the system that controls everything that is meant to happen automatically in the body – your heartbeat, digestion, circulation, immune system etc. As you can imagine this had a pretty devastating effect on my life – I literally couldn't walk down the street, I slept for sixteen hours a day, was in chronic pain, had blackouts, never-ending heart palpitations, unbearable stomach issues, constant headaches and the list goes on. It was anything but fun and I was bedridden ninety-five per cent of the time. Life as I knew it was put on hold.

Being this ill was a bigger challenge then I could ever have imagined. Up until this point I'd always been really healthy and so I really never saw it coming. At the time I was just nineteen and had been spending my summer in Paris, pursuing a career in modelling and having the best time. Going from that to a hospital bed within the space of just a few weeks really shook me and as my hospital trips got longer and longer and doctor after doctor ran out of suggestions as to what was wrong with me, I really fell apart. It took four months of hospital visits and hundreds of tests to finally get a diagnosis, and I still remember that huge sense of relief when my wonderful doctor gave my illness a name. At the very least people could no longer tell me it was psychological!

The thing was that even though my illness now had a name, this didn't really make anything much better, and certainly not as much as I thought it would. I was put on a whole series of different drugs and steroids, some of which gave me new symptoms and none of which really helped. I was still essentially bed-bound, which created a huge sense of isolation, and my confidence and self-esteem vanished. It felt impossible to keep up with any friends. This was partly because of a lack of energy and a desire to sleep all the time, but it was also because I was too embarrassed to tell anyone what was really happening. I didn't want everyone to look at me like a sick person and I felt like a total alien, so different from everyone else that I just couldn't really relate to them.

In January 2012 I decided to try and be a 'normal' person and take a trip with my boyfriend. We went to Marrakesh, but the trip in some ways was a total disaster and I ended up being brought home, semi-conscious, in a wheelchair. Of course in lots of ways this wasn't ideal, but it was actually exactly what I needed as it woke me up to what was really happening to me. It became clear that it was my responsibility to change my situation. I could no longer rely on my doctors and I had to find a way to get my life back. So I spent the next week researching holistic, natural approaches to healing, which is what led me to change my diet.

After a lot of Googling I came across some incredibly inspirational people, in particular a woman in the US called Kris Carr, who overnight changed my life. She had changed her diet to manage her cancer and had written a wonderful book all about it, so I ordered the book and immediately realised that if she could come back from that I could absolutely come back from where I was. So, overnight I started a wholefoods, plant-based diet and gave up all meat, dairy, sugar, gluten, anything processed and all chemicals and additives. As you can imagine it was a really difficult change for someone who had never eaten fruit or vegetables before, let alone quinoa, buckwheat and chia seeds! I'll never forget the looks on my family's faces when I told them I was becoming a gluten-free vegan – I don't think I've ever seen people so surprised and confused. I'm not sure they believed I'd last a day but I was very determined to really give it a try. The only problem was I didn't have a clue what to eat!

HEALING FOOD

I was all ready to go with my healthy eating healing regime until it suddenly occurred to me that not only did I not know what to eat, but I also couldn't cook! I mean I could boil pasta and scramble a couple of eggs, but that was really about it. Nonetheless I really wanted to try this new way of life, so for the next three months or so I literally ate the same thing every day. Breakfast was banana and blueberry porridge, with the fruit added in right at the beginning to ensure it fully disintegrated (little did I know that this method actually gives more flavour). Lunch was buckwheat toast with mashed avocado and roasted tomatoes: totally delicious but a little repetitive every day! And dinner was brown rice pasta with some form of veggie sauce.

As you can imagine I was suffering from some serious food envy as everyone around me tucked into a fantastic array of different foods and I continued with the same meals day after day. Yet something amazing was happening: I was starting to feel better! My symptoms were lessening and my energy was returning – it was just the most incredible feeling. It was slow, but it was unbelievably exciting and so encouraging. It really inspired me to get more into what I was doing and that's where my blog, Deliciously Ella, came in. I thought that if I kept a blog and promised myself that I'd try three new recipes a week, then I would start really loving this new way of cooking, which is exactly what happened.

I had some funny reactions from people when I told them I was starting a food blog, mostly with people saying 'But you don't cook' – which up

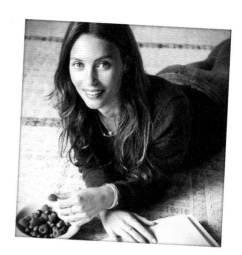

until that point was absolutely true. In fact, the first time I offered to cook for my boyfriend he even had dinner before coming over. So I decided to keep the blog private but promised after twenty posts that I'd show it to a couple of friends, and it all just grew from there. As my readership slowly grew, so did my knowledge and my confidence in cooking in a completely new way, and eighteen months later the blog had had over five million hits, which was quite a surreal feeling. Readers even started to get in touch to tell me how my recipes had changed *their* life, which was incredibly inspiring. In fact, I've decided to share some of my favourite comments in the book.

Anyway, as if all that wasn't exciting enough, something even more incredible had happened – I felt healed! My healthy eating adventure had really worked and in less than two years I was off all the medication I should have been on for life. It felt like a miracle: my symptoms had all but disappeared and my self-esteem was rebuilt, all thanks to the goodness of plants. It was amazing. I felt free and truly like myself again.

The decision to change my diet really was single-handedly the best thing I've ever done. It allowed me to take control of my illness and get my life back, which was so empowering. It's been quite a journey and I've learnt so much, which is why I wanted to write this book – so that I could share all my findings with you. It's my way of turning a negative into a positive. I know how daunting healthy food can be and I want to make it easy for you.

A WORLD OF GOODNESS

As I have discovered there are ways of making all your favourite foods healthy and delicious – hello brownies, pizza and ice cream – it's just a question of learning how, and I'm going to share all the tricks I've learnt with you here. I also want to emphasise that I'm not a chef, I'm a cook and everything comes from experiments in my own kitchen, which I hope will make it seem even more accessible to you.

It took me about six months to really get the hang of cooking this way and every time I tried a new recipe I couldn't believe how well it worked. There were two things that really stood out. Firstly, that it was all really easy. I mean seriously easy. I couldn't believe that we weren't all enjoying the simplicity of this way of cooking. The other thing I was really surprised about was that it was all so incredibly quick to make, which I especially loved. I'm not a fan of spending hours cooking – it always seemed a little crazy to me to spend five hours cooking one meal! But I was turning round insanely delicious dinner parties, which all my friends loved, in just half an hour or so. They'd all be so excited and impressed by what I was serving, so much so that I almost felt like I was cheating as it had been so straightforward to prepare. My other favourite thing was that I was whipping up awesome weekday suppers for one in just ten minutes. I loved coming home at the end of the day knowing I was going to eat a sumptuous, insanely nutritious feast!

I know this kind of plant-based, wholefood living does has some slightly negative stereotypes attached to it, which I absolutely fell for too. I mean I would never have believed you if you'd told me five years ago that today I'd be a gluten-free vegan! But I really hope that this book will change your perceptions, just as mine have changed along the way. I hope that my recipes will show you that healthy food is so much more than bland salads, boiled veggies and iceberg lettuce. It's gooey sweet potato brownies, carrot cake with caramel icing, silky chocolate mousse, beautiful rainbow salads with creamy dressings, perfectly seasoned roasted veg with homemade pesto, courgette noodles with avocado cream, sweet potato fries and spicy coconut curries.

All my recipes are both gluten-free and plant-based, as well as refined sugar-free, but I promise you that I absolutely haven't written this with the intention of converting you all to veganism. I'm not a huge fan of the word vegan anyway, as you can also be a very unhealthy vegan. Instead I'm all about whole, natural foods that nourish your body. I'm really not here to point fingers though or encourage feelings of guilt, and I'm absolutely not expecting you to start eating entirely this way tomorrow. Instead this book is meant to be flexible and adaptable, it's just about showing how amazingly easy and delicious plants can be so that we can all start enjoying more of them. However, you don't have to eat this way all the time. You can make it work for you, adding cheese to your baked sweet potato, a side of salmon to your quinoa, some yoghurt to your smoothie or some milk to your tea – that's just not a problem. As long as you're loving your plants I'm happy!

A NEW WAY OF EATING

My biggest advice would be to start making small changes first, just adding in one new serving of fruit or veg a day is an amazing way to start. For example some sweet potato wedges or guacamole make a delicious addition to any meal and they're so easy to make. Whizzing up a smoothie in the morning is incredible too as it always starts you off on the right track for a positive day, while giving you an abundance of goodness and making you glow from the inside out!

The other thing that I want to stress is that the Deliciously Ella lifestyle is about counting goodness not calories. We're not focusing on dieting and deprivation here, which I know are things often associated with healthy eating. Instead I'm hoping that this book might help to change your mindset in the way that it did for me, so that we can all celebrate amazing food and feel incredible about ourselves at the same time. We all get sweet cravings, it's completely normal, and I'm really not here to say that you shouldn't have that something sweet. I'm simply saying that there are amazing, natural alternatives which taste just as good – if not better – than the processed, sugar-laden desserts everyone is used to and they'll make you feel so much better too. With any luck I can also dispel myths that eating things like avocados and almonds will make you fat too. Everything you see in here is so amazingly good for you that you really can and should eat as much of these things as you like as your body absolutely loves them and they'll energise you more than you can imagine.

I love the way I eat now. It's become an incredible new way of life and I'm honestly happier then I've ever been. I feel fantastic and everything tastes better too; my taste buds are so much stronger and I'd take a batch of sweet potato brownies over pick 'n' mix any day! I hope my book helps you fall in love with natural food in the way that I have and that through cooking my food and trying new things you will feel amazing too.

Ella x

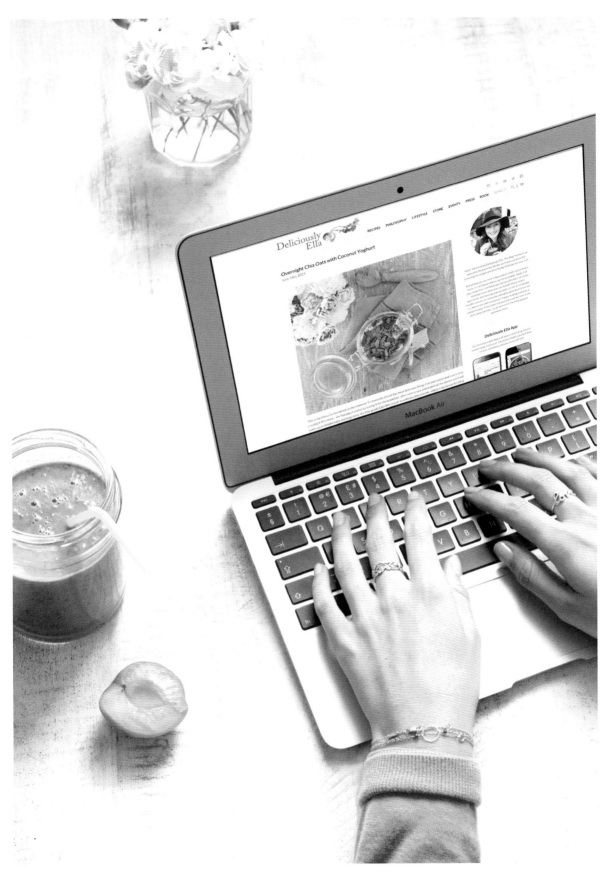

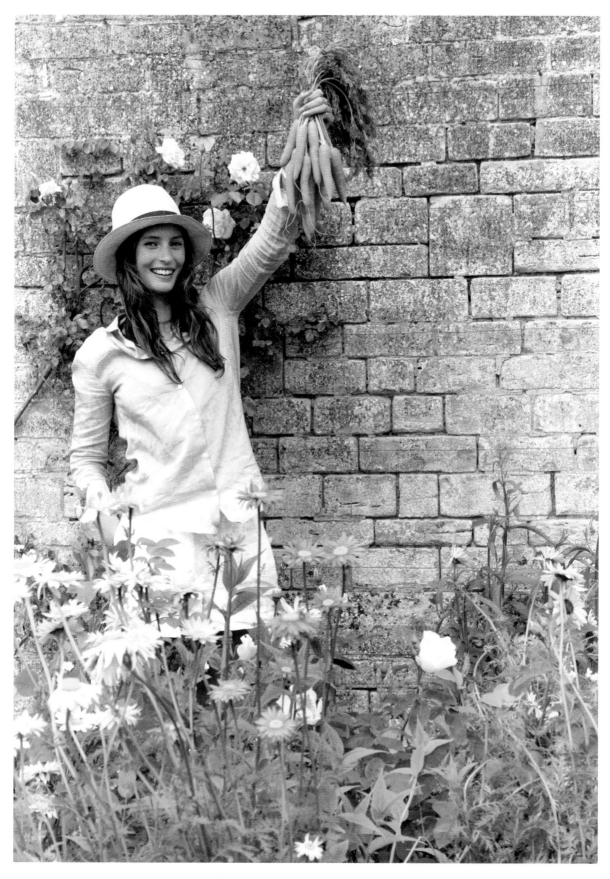

GETTING STARTED

One of the questions I get asked most is how you can eat this way if you're busy, to which the answer is: by being organised. I know it might sound really boring, but stocking your pantry is an essential part of eating well as it means that whatever happens you can always whip up something delicious, even with very basic ingredients. I keep a collection of staple items in my cupboards so that I'm never stuck and it really makes eating this way so easy. I normally order all these basics online every couple of months to make sure that I always have them.

You'll find as you go through the book that almost all of the recipes include a selection of the ingredients discussed in this chapter. I find it so annoying when recipes call for random, hard-to-find ingredients, which you buy and then never use again. I've tried to consistently use the same basics, which means that you can do one shop and then you'll be good to go for every recipe – all you need to do is buy the fresh fruits and veggies. It may seem pricey when you first buy everything, but trust me, it's so worth it, as your food will taste better than ever, and actually over time it's not expensive as you'll only ever be spending a few pounds on fresh produce for your day-to-day meals.

There are a few awesome things that you can make from scratch yourself too, so I've included the recipes for them in this chapter in order to get you started. Things like nut butters, dairy-free milks, apple purée, home-made salts and an easy vegetable stock.

MY KITCHEN ESSENTIALS

Having these core ingredients in the cupboard makes meals extra delicious and it's always nice to be eating meals where almost everything is made from scratch, as you know it's all packed with goodness. These ingredients played a huge role in my healing processes and really helped me learn to love clean, natural food, so once you're using all of these you'll see amazing things happen too! I've given a little information on each of the ingredients so hopefully you'll understand why I love them so much and when to use them, so that you can get creative in your kitchen!

APPLE CIDER VINEGAR

Apple cider vinegar is an awesome ingredient. It's a great alternative to balsamic vinegar as it is very alkalinising and amazing for digestive issues. If you're having digestive issues you can take a shot of it before every meal, which will do wonders, but I do have to warn you that it isn't the most delicious thing on its own! I normally use it in salad dressings or to add flavour to dips, sauces and grains. It has a light, tangy flavour that echoes lemons or limes, so it's a great alternative for those too if you don't have them in the house.

COCONUT MILK

Coconut milk is one of the most delicious things ever. I just love how insanely creamy it is, which means that it makes the best addition to anything where you'd normally want to use cow's milk or cream. I use it most in my porridge, smoothies and baking, but I also add it to dishes like risotto to make them extra creamy. It has a pretty mild flavour – the coconut taste doesn't come through as much as it does in coconut oil or creamed coconut – so you can get all the benefits of the awesome texture without making your savoury dishes taste of coconut. Coconut cream is different to coconut milk, though. Coconut cream is totally solid and has no liquid at all, whereas coconut milk is runny.

COCONUT OIL

Another important member of the coconut family is coconut oil, one of the most versatile ingredients ever and one of my all-time favourites. I swear you can use it for basically anything from beauty and hair care to baking and cooking. It's great as an alternative to olive oil for roasting your veggies if you're after a more intense flavour, or added into your smoothie for an extra boost of energy. If you're allergic to nuts, it's a great nut butter replacement in smoothies too, as it creates the same smooth, creamy texture. I also use it to line all my tins when I'm baking cakes, muffins or bread, as well as stirring it into my porridge for extra creaminess. Whilst it is high in fat, the fat is all really good for you and it's especially important for glowing skin!

FRESH FRUIT

There are a few fresh items that I always buy at the beginning of every week so that even if I'm too busy to buy fresh food for a few days, I know there's always something good to eat. For me the staples are bananas, apples, lemons, limes and frozen berries. I buy frozen organic berries in bulk, which are much cheaper than fresh berries except when they're in season, so that I can always add them to my smoothies. I buy bananas for the same reason; I love my smoothies and they're normally the basis of them. Plus bananas mashed with almond butter and a sprinkling of salt on

crackers or my superfood bread is the best snack or three-minute dinner ever. Apples I buy as they're a great snack and are delicious juiced. And the lemons and limes are to spice up my food – even the blandest meal can be made a million times more delicious with a drizzling of fresh lemon or lime juice. I mean, is there anything better than a mashed avocado with fresh lime juice and salt or home-made hummus? Neither of those have complicated ingredients and can be whipped up in five minutes, as long as you have my list of essentials in your house.

GLUTEN-FREE FLOURS

Gluten-free flour is a really important staple. I'm not talking about the refined, ready-mixed stuff, but pure buckwheat, quinoa and brown rice flours. Just to sort out any confusion, buckwheat doesn't actually contain any wheat or gluten – the name is totally misleading – but it's actually super-healthy and totally uncontaminated by gluten. Brown rice and buckwheat flours are absolutely interchangeable; both have a pretty mild flavour that works equally well in sweet and savoury baking. Quinoa flour has a more bitter flavour that lends itself really well to savoury food, but to be honest, it's really not very nice in baking unless you use industrial quantities of sweetener! These flours are easy to find online or at any health-food shop.

GLUTEN-FREE PASTA

As with gluten-free flour, I'm not talking about corn or white rice pasta here, but quinoa or brown rice pasta. If you're not allergic to gluten, then spelt is a good option too. Spelt is an ancient strain of gluten that is much less refined and processed, so most people tolerate it much better than wheat. I've never tried spelt pasta though, as I can't eat gluten, so I can't one hundred per cent vouch for it tasting amazing, but I've only ever heard positive reviews! Brown rice and quinoa pasta are both totally delicious though and I promise you really won't realise that there's any difference to normal pasta – the taste and texture are exactly the same, especially if you're using a delicious sauce! I like to keep these in the house so that I can always whip up a filling meal in ten minutes. There's a great recipe for my Ten-Minute Tomato Pasta later on in the book too (page 131)!

GRAINS

I've dedicated a whole chapter to Grains (page 29) so you'll get so much more info on all of them specifically there, but for now I just want to share my staples, which are brown rice, quinoa, buckwheat and oats. I have huge jars of all four of them in my kitchen so that I never run out. It means that if I need a speedy meal, I can always make something substantial with one of them as the base, like my coconut porridge. I also try to make a big batch of either brown rice, quinoa or buckwheat every week so that I can just warm one up with some tahini, tamari and lime or lemon juice plus a tin of beans and a mashed avocado for an amazing five-minute meal. Oats and brown rice are the easiest to get hold of as they're found in all supermarkets, but most supermarkets now sell quinoa too, which is great. For buckwheat, you normally need either a health-food shop or an online stockist.

HERBS AND SPICES

Herbs and spices are absolutely vital in any kitchen as they make food come alive; without them life is pretty boring! My essentials are some mixed herbs or herbes de Provence, cinnamon, turmeric, paprika, cumin and chilli flakes – with those in your cupboards you really can't go wrong. I use a mix of all of them on absolutely everything and it instantly adds layers of deep flavours to even the simplest dishes. It's really easy to keep your own fresh herbs too, they tend to have more flavour and end up being much cheaper. Basil,

rosemary, thyme and mint are all grown really easily on windowsills or in patio pots. I like having fresh ginger too and garlic as they also add amazing flavour and they're easy to get from any supermarket. I don't eat onion though, which you may notice as you go through the book; it just doesn't agree with my stomach, but please feel free to add it to any recipe if you're an onion lover!

MEDJOOL DATES

Medjool dates are totally heavenly; again I've given them lots of attention in the Fruit section (page 173) so I won't overload you with information here – except to say that I think these are the best food on earth! As you'll discover later, they're the most magical ingredient to bake with, but they're also an amazing snack, which is why I like to keep them in my house. They're so insanely sweet and taste a lot like caramel, so if I'm after something sweet and don't want to start cooking, then I'll enjoy a handful of these beauties. My favourite thing to do is to remove the stone and then fill each one with a teaspoon of nut butter; trust me on this one, it's one of the best things you'll ever eat. Now, Medjool dates are more expensive than normal dates, but they're so worth the price difference as they're so much softer and sweeter. They're also more delicious and much easier to cook with, especially when they're used to stick the mix together, as in all the raw desserts and snacks later in the book. Sadly, you'll find that these recipes won't always turn out quite right if you use the dried dates as they are simply not sticky enough.

NUTS

As with the grains, I've dedicated a whole chapter to Nuts and Seeds (page 65), so you'll get more specific information there on each nut, how it tastes and what it works best in, but for now I'd like to tell you a little bit about why they should be a pantry staple. Not only do they taste amazing and so make great little snack bowls, but in five minutes you can also whip up an awesome raw sweet treat using essentially just dates and nuts! My favourite is the recipe for my Raw Brownies (page 89), which have just three ingredients – nuts, dates and raw cacao – and they taste so insanely good that you'll be skipping round your kitchen! The other thing is that having these ingredients, which allow you to create something so delicious in such a short time, means you're way less likely to start snacking on the less healthy things as you won't be craving them, which means your taste buds and your tummy will both be happy!

NUT BUTTERS

Whilst I love nuts – they're great – I absolutely adore nut butters. They're one of the best creations ever. I can, and often do, sit with a teaspoon and eat a whole jar at once! Each bite is just so insanely creamy, nicely sweet, yet not sickly and so tasty. Obviously they taste amazing with a spoon, but they also have a lot of other uses, which is why they're included in my essentials list. A spoonful of nut butter is a great addition to any quick snack or breakfast as it adds great flavour, a delicious texture and a whole lot of goodness with

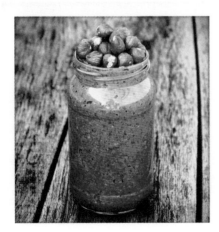

tons of plant protein, amazing fats and vitamins that will really boost your energy levels. I add a spoonful of almond butter to my smoothie every morning and always add some to my porridge too. In the afternoon, I often snack on things like mashed banana with almond butter, dates stuffed with nut butter or sliced apple dipped into nut butter – all so delicious and so easy to make with almost no mess to clean up afterwards! The bigger supermarkets stock nut butters, as do all health-food shops and tons of online shops.

OLIVE OIL

There are few things that make me happier than a bottle of really good, organic, extra virgin olive oil. I might sound all fancy with my requirement that the oil is such a high standard, but trust me on this one, it makes the world of difference and if you're going to splurge on one thing, do it on olive oil! You can even have two different bottles, one pretty standard one to use on your veggies whilst you cook them and then one amazing one to add at the end so that you can really enjoy it. Good olive oil really does have such a strong flavour and such a beautifully smooth, rich texture that enhances the taste of absolutely everything. You can use it in the most conventional ways to liven up salads, but you can also drizzle it over dishes like risottos, stir it into your grains as they finish cooking or mix it into mashed avocado to add another layer of awesomeness to your creation! The easiest place to buy great olive oil is either in a farmers' market, online or at a lovely deli; supermarket olive oil should really just be used to cook with as it doesn't have the real flavour.

PULSES

So you'll learn a lot more about pulses in the Beans and Pulses chapter (page 97), but they're an important part of my pantry for the same reasons as grains – they add instant substance to any meal. The thing that really makes them stand out though, is the fact that they can be ready in a minute or two. I always have several tins of black beans, chickpeas and lentils in my cupboard so that all I have to do is open the can, drain the water and then I'm good to go – it's that easy! The chickpeas are essential so that I can whip up an awesome bowl of hummus in a couple of minutes too, which immediately makes any meal more exciting and more energising. All pulses are amazingly energising though as they're so full of B vitamins, protein and iron, which are all essential for a healthy body and happy mind!

RAW CACAO POWDER

Raw cacao powder is one of my all-time favourite ingredients; I really don't know what I would do without it. It's one of the few things that I really crave too – I just can't get enough of its rich, chocolaty goodness. So what's the difference between raw cacao powder and the cocoa powder you buy in the supermarkets? Raw cacao is the unprocessed version; it's simply a ground-down version of the cacao bean. Cocoa, on the other hand, has been processed and refined so almost all the goodness is gone and it doesn't taste half as good either! Raw cacao is so much richer and stronger – so you need less of it to create the same flavour – plus it's packed with antioxidants, vitamins and minerals so you really can eat chocolate in the knowledge that it's actually good for you! Don't be put off by the price of the raw cacao either, as it ends up being cheaper than nice cocoa as you need so much less of it. You'll need just a few tablespoons of raw cacao for every box of cocoa – it's awesome!

SEEDS

While seeds can't make up the basis of a meal in the way that grains and beans can, they're a great thing to have around as they add real texture to anything, making your meal much more exciting, whilst also boosting its levels of goodness. I love sprinkling sunflower and pumpkin seeds on just about anything from salads, to curries, to dips, to pasta dishes and, of course, over my mashed avocado! The other magic seeds that I like to keep around are chia seeds and you'll learn more about their incredible qualities later (page 70), but they're pretty essential for healthy baking, plus they're powerhouses of nutrition and they don't taste of anything, so you can mix them into whatever you're eating to get a great dose of protein, calcium, fibre and omega-3s.

SWEETENERS

My go-to sweeteners are pure maple syrup and honey; both are totally delicious and are essential for so many dishes, from pancakes and waffles to blueberry muffins, key lime pie and sweet potato brownies. I drizzle raw honey over my toast too and sometimes add it to my green smoothie if it's a little too green for my liking that day! The important thing to watch out for when you buy maple syrup is that it really is one hundred per cent maple syrup because a lot of them are ten per cent maple syrup and ninety per cent weird additives, sweeteners and preservatives – always read the label! Honey is a more complicated subject. There are so many different varieties and it's much less obvious which ones are good and which ones are bad. I prefer buying raw honey, which you can find pretty easily from places like Holland & Barrett. It's not super expensive and has the strongest, most amazing taste. It's normally £2 to £3 a jar, so much better value than Manuka honey, which can come closer to £20 a jar! I tend to avoid the very cheap squeezy honeys that they sell in supermarkets as they can be quite processed and instead try to find markets that sell local honey if I don't have any of my raw honey.

TAHINI

Tahini is a pretty wondrous ingredient. It's made from ground sesame seeds, which form a thick paste, just like peanut butter. It's more savoury than nut butter though, and whilst I love it mixed into various dishes, I don't love it on its own, so unlike my nut butter I won't sit and eat the whole thing with a spoon! I find it's too savoury for smoothies or sweet things, but it's incredible stirred into grains, rubbed into kale, blended into dips or mixed with olive oil and apple cider vinegar for an awesome salad dressing. It adds such a rich flavour and creamy texture to whatever you pair it with, which automatically enhances your creation, making it much more exciting. Of course it's the key ingredient in hummus too and you'll find it in all my various hummus recipes on page 102. Sesame seeds are also full of goodness, particularly calcium, B vitamins, magnesium and iron, so they're a great thing to add to your diet.

TAMARI AND MISO PASTE

If you're going to buy just a handful of ingredients, I would so recommend including either some tamari or miso paste. Both are made from fermented soy beans: tamari is a liquid version and miso paste is, of course, a paste, so it's much thicker and a little richer. They have the same flavour though. To avoid any confusion about tamari versus soy sauce, I should quickly say that they're almost identical, except that tamari is gluten-free (and normally free of funny additives too), which is why I use it, but you can use soy sauce in any of the recipes that call for tamari if you prefer. I use tamari and miso paste interchangeably to add a salty flavour, which is especially great if you're trying to cut down your salt intake. Both really work to enhance all the existing flavours, without drastically altering them. I add one or the other to almost everything to make my dishes more interesting.

TOMATO PURÉE AND TINS OF TOMATOES

Neither tomato purée nor tins of tomatoes are especially exotic or exciting, so I won't go into too much detail here except to say that both are amazing things to keep stocked in your cupboards for those days that you need to quickly rustle something up with almost no ingredients. Recipes like my Ten-Minute Tomato Pasta (page 131) are life savers for busy, hungry days and it really helps if you already have the tomato purée in your kitchen. Likewise, you can use the tinned tomatoes to make easy curries and stews with whatever you have lying around, then just add some brown rice seasoned with tamari and you're good to go! With both, just check the ingredients before you buy them that there are no added preservatives and sugars as there sometimes are with these items. Plus, tomatoes are amazingly good for us as they're packed with antioxidants, which are so important for beautiful skin!

VEGETABLES

Since this is a plant-based cookbook, you'll find information on different veggies on almost every page, but I just wanted to share with you the key veggies that I keep in my kitchen at all times as these are the ones that I use every day – the others I buy as and when I need them. For me, the essentials are leafy greens in the form of spinach and kale, tomatoes, avocados and cucumbers. The leafy greens I eat every day in some form. I normally add spinach to my morning smoothie and eat some kale salad as a side with either lunch or dinner. The cucumbers I juice in batches every couple of days to use as the base of my smoothies. The avocados are there just because I'm totally addicted to them and can't go a day without eating at least one, while the tomatoes are always handy as they go with just about anything! Having a handful of veggies like this means that there's always something you can eat, whether it's a kale salad marinated with tahini and tamari (page 153) and served with a side of brown rice and beans or mashed avocado with sliced tomato on Superfood Bread (page 80), I know there's always a delicious option waiting for me.

HOME-MADE SALTS

These salts are the best way to instantly add a mix of delicious flavours to whatever you're cooking. The Chilli Salt adds a wonderful fiery, spicy touch that really livens up any vegetable, grain or bean, while the Herb Salt adds a subtler range of flavours, with its delicious mix of thyme, rosemary, cumin and lemon, which together enhance all the natural flavours of your meal.

CHILLI SALT

Fills 1 x 60g salt grinder

20g rock salt

3g black peppercorns

2 tablespoons paprika

1 tablespoon chilli flakes

Simply mix the rock salt, pepper, paprika and chilli flakes in bowl and then pour them into your salt grinder.

HERB SALT

Fills 1 x 60g salt grinder

20g fresh rosemary sprigs

20g fresh thyme sprigs

zest of 1 large lemon

1 tablespoon whole cumin seeds

20g rock salt

Preheat the oven to 220°C (fan 200°C).

Place the rosemary and thyme leaves on a baking tray (you don't need to add any oil) and bake for about 8 minutes, until the herbs are completely dry.

Once the rosemary and thyme are dry, remove them from the oven and allow them to cool.

Place the lemon zest on a baking tray and bake for about 2 minutes, until it's also dry.

Finally, mix the baked herbs, lemon zest, cumin and rock salt in a bowl before pouring it into your salt grinder.

APPLE PURÉE

As you go through the book, you'll see that I use apple purée all the time, partly because it's delicious and partly because it's such a diverse ingredient, which works so well in cooking, especially baking. It does two particularly awesome things – firstly, it adds sweetness to whatever you're cooking in a very natural way and secondly, it works as the perfect egg replacement to stick everything together. I love using it on its own as a spread, though it tastes especially amazing stirred into porridge (page 57) or piled onto pancakes (page 163) or waffles (page 183).

makes 1 large jar

20 red apples

optional: 3 tablespoons date syrup (maple syrup also works)

optional: 1 tablespoon ground cinnamon

Peel the apples and chop them into bite-sized pieces, discarding the core.

Place all the apple pieces in a large saucepan and cover the bottom with a couple of centimetres of water.

Allow the apples to cook for about 40 minutes, until they're very soft.

At this point, drain any remaining water and add the apples to a blender or a food processor with the date syrup and cinnamon, if you're using them, and blend until smooth and creamy.

Store in an airtight container in the fridge – it will stay fresh for about 5 days.

Top tip

This only stays fresh for about 5 days, so if you make more than you're going to use, then freeze the rest.

DAIRY-FREE MILKS

Making dairy-free milks is actually way simpler then you'd imagine, and they honestly do taste really good!

Almond milk is my favourite of the three milks here as it's the creamiest and richest. You can use the almond milk recipe for any nut though, not just almonds; brazil nuts and cashews make wonderful milk too.

Oat milk is quicker and much less expensive to make than almond milk though, which makes it a great option – plus it works well if you're allergic to nuts. It's lovely and sweet too, I have to admit that it does bear a slight resemblance to liquid porridge, but that doesn't mean it's not delicious!

Rice milk doesn't really compare to almond or oat milk in texture or taste sadly, but if you can't eat nuts or oats, then it works well in any of the recipes. It does need some sweetening though as it's not naturally as flavoursome, and it's much runnier too! It's really inexpensive though and very easy to make.

All three last about 5 days in the fridge. Just be sure to keep them in an airtight container; an old water bottle will work perfectly if you don't have any glass bottles to hand. They will separate as you store them, so just give them a good shake before you pour the milk out.

ALMOND MILK
makes 1 litre

1 mug blanched almonds (200g)
optional: 2 teaspoons ground cinnamon
optional: handful of pitted Medjool dates or a
  couple of spoonfuls of date or maple syrup

Soak the almonds for at least 6 hours or overnight in a bowl of water. This process is absolutely essential.

Drain the nuts and add them to a blender with 3 mugs (900ml) fresh water. Blend it all for a minute or two until smooth milk forms; if you want your milk a little runnier, add more water.

Place a jelly bag strainer on the top of a jug and pour the milk through it.

Once the bag is partially drained, squeeze the rest of the liquid out with your hands.

If you're using the cinnamon, dates or syrup, blend the milk with these in the blender.

BROWN RICE MILK
makes 1 litre

⅓ mug brown rice (90g)
2 tablespoons maple syrup or honey
1 teaspoon ground cinnamon

Put the rice in a saucepan with 1½ mugs (450ml) water. Bring the pan to the boil and let it bubble for 5 minutes or so, then simmer for about 45 minutes, covered, until the rice is soft, but not soggy, and all the water has evaporated. You'll need to stir the rice and make sure the rice never runs out of water until it is done.

Blend the cooled rice with 3 mugs of water, the maple syrup or honey and cinnamon, until smooth.

Pour the blended brown rice mix through a fine sieve to sieve out any grit before serving.

OAT MILK
makes 1 litre

1 mug oats (120g)
optional: 1-2 tablespoons sweetener (I use honey
  or maple syrup)

Soak the oats in cold water for about 30 minutes.

Rinse and drain the oats before placing them into a blender with 3 mugs (900ml) fresh water. Blend for about 30 seconds until smooth.

Pour the blended oat mix through a fine sieve, using a wooden spoon to push it through. Discard the pulp.

Stir the sweetener into the milk, if you're using it, and then place the milk back into the blender and blend again.

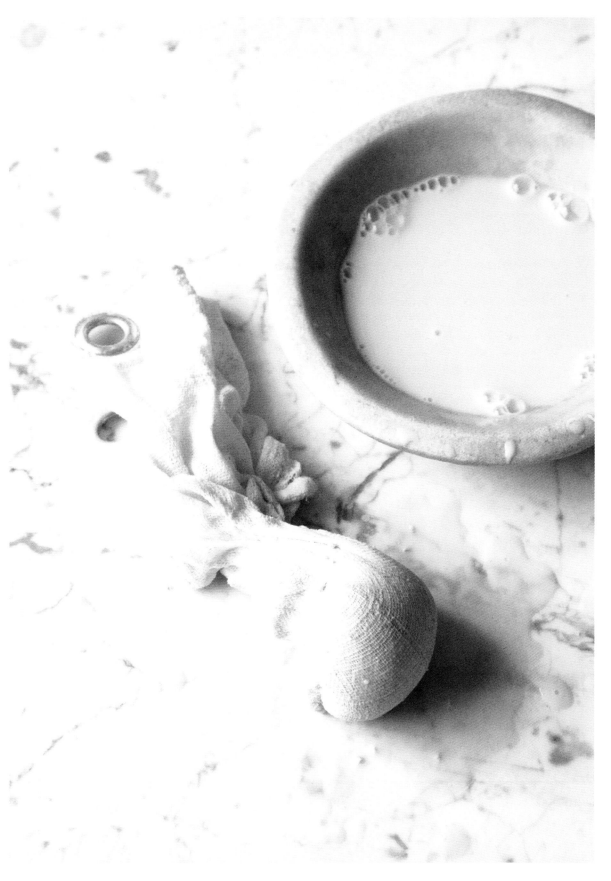

THE EQUIPMENT THAT I CAN'T LIVE WITHOUT

There are a couple of pieces of equipment that are totally essential to this lifestyle. You'll need a food processor, a blender and a juicer to make the vast majority of these recipes, but I promise that's it. Other than these three things, you really don't need anything else outside of your standard kitchen equipment – just simple things like knives, pots, pans, a grater, chopping board, jelly bag, sieve and steamer.

A food processor breaks down whatever you put into it. They're incredibly strong and can turn a solid into a liquid very easily, which is pretty cool! Unlike a blender, they don't need liquid to run, but the end result isn't quite as smooth so you can't make your smoothies in a processor. Instead, it's used to make things like hummus and pesto, to crush nuts and to make raw desserts.

A blender needs liquid to run and creates an incredibly smooth product, so it's used to make soups and smoothies.

A juicer is a great investment, but if you're choosing what to buy first, start with the processor and blender as these are used in so many different recipes, whereas a juicer is only used to make juices, which is great, but it's not multi-purpose so it's less essential.

THE BRANDS I USE AND LOVE

FOOD PROCESSOR

Magimix food processors are the best food processors ever. Yes, they are expensive, but it's a life-long investment and so worth it – you can make literally anything in them! My mum and all her friends are still using the ones that they were given as wedding presents, so they really do last.

BLENDER

I use a Vitamix blender. Again, they are pretty pricey (much more so than the Magimix), but if

you're going to use it every day, then it's worth the investment as they are amazing. They are so powerful, which means that they make the smoothest, creamiest smoothies and can handle absolutely anything that you throw into the mix. If you're not already a total health food and smoothie fanatic and are looking for something to ease you in, then there are some other great companies that do good blenders for a lot less.

If you're looking for a less expensive blender, Philips makes really good ones for about £80, which will do everything that you need. Again, it may seem like a lot, but the blenders that cost less aren't that strong, which means that they can't break down things like nuts, dates and spinach into a smooth drink, which is essential – trust me, strands of spinach do not taste good in between sips of mango and banana! Plus the more you spend now, the longer it will last, so the less you'll have to spend in the future.

Tribest Personal Blender and Nutribullets are amazing personal blenders. They're really strong and absolutely tiny in comparison to the Philips or Vitamix. The blender part also detaches so that you can take it on the go with you, which is great. Both cost about £100 and are great options for travelling or if you know you're only ever going to be making smoothies for one.

JUICER

Magimix and Sage both make great juicers, which are very easy to wash up! This is honestly my biggest consideration when buying a juicer as even the best of them are a nightmare to get clean as there are several different parts and the pulp always gets stuck in some of it.

JELLY BAG

The last thing you'll need that isn't totally standard is a jelly bag as it's essential for making nut milk. Don't worry though, these are really cheap and easy to find as they're normally used for making jams or jellies so they're always stocked in places like John Lewis or online from places like Amazon. Each bag costs somewhere between £1 and £3 and they last for ages. I normally rinse mine after I use it and then, after a couple of uses, I'll put it into the washing machine for a proper clean.

SIEVE

To make oat milk or rice milk, you'll also need a fine sieve, but any old sieve works great – you don't need anything fancy.

I know I've just thrown a lot of information at you really quickly and I hope it doesn't seem too overwhelming! Hopefully as you go through the book you'll see that the things I've talked about here really are so easy to use and, most importantly, they're used over and over again so you should get to grips with them really quickly! I know I was a little overwhelmed when I first started my adventure into healthy eating, so I do totally understand the feeling, but it will get easier! Plus, the learning is pretty fun and it's ongoing forever – I'm still learning now and I'm always finding cool new ingredients to try and interesting new ways of cooking!

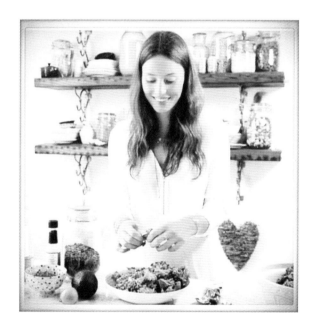

ALMOND BUTTER

Almond butter is one of my staples and I use it every day. It just has the most beautifully creamy texture and an amazing rich, nutty flavour. I love adding it to my smoothies to thicken them up and it's also amazing stirred into my Creamy Coconut Porridge (page 57) and, of course, eaten straight from the jar with a spoon! It's amazing skin food too as it's bursting with vitamin E, which is essential for a glowing complexion. I like roasting my nuts first as this allows them to blend more easily, while also enhancing their flavour, but if you prefer you can skip this step. You can also use any other nut to make nut butter using the same process.

makes 1 large jar
2 mugs almonds (400g)
sprinkling of salt

Preheat the oven to 200°C (fan 180°C).

Roast the almonds for about 10 minutes, then remove them and allow them to cool for a few minutes.

Place the nuts in a food processor and blend for about 15 minutes with the salt until smooth and creamy. During this time, you might need to scrape the nuts off the side of the processor once or twice.

Store in an airtight container at room temperature for up to a week.

Top tip
You really need a strong food processor for this recipe as otherwise it won't get really smooth and creamy.

MEDJOOL DATES STUFFED WITH NUT BUTTER

This may not be the most complicated recipe in the book, in fact it may well be the simplest, but that doesn't mean it's not the best! This is my go-to snack when I'm hungry and feeling lazy. It's sweet and satisfying and oh-so-delicious. The caramel-like dates complement the creamy almond butter so well – it's a match made in heaven.

makes 12 dates
12 Medjool dates
12 teaspoons nut butter (I like almond butter best – see recipe on this page)
optional: a sprinkling of raw cacao powder

Peel the dates open, without totally cutting them in half, and remove the stones.

Place a small teaspoon of nut butter and a sprinkling of cacao powder where the stone was and push the two halves of the date together again.

Place the stuffed dates in the fridge to firm up for about an hour and then enjoy.

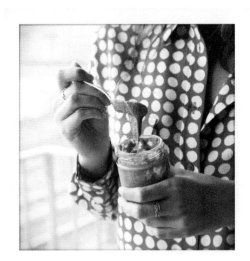

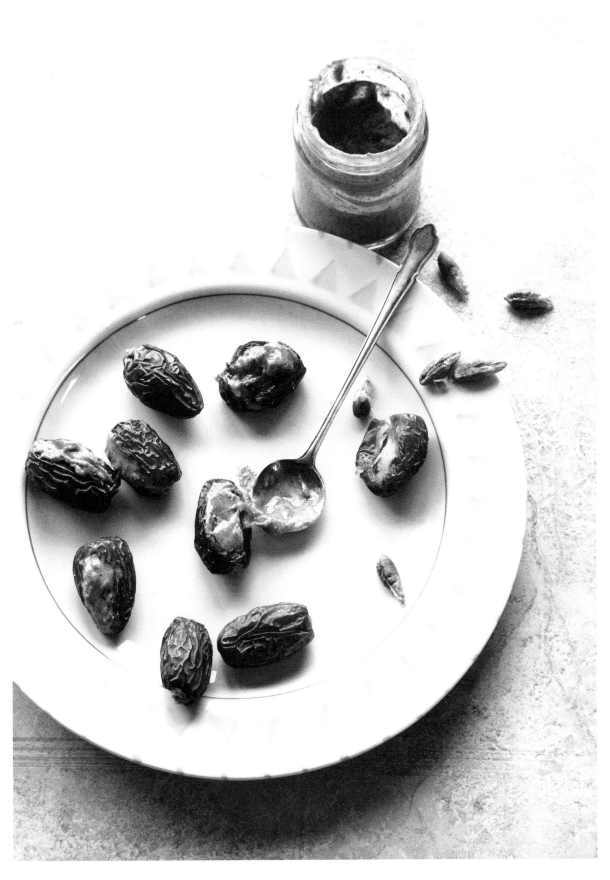

HOW TO COOK GRAINS

You'll learn much more about grains in the Grains chapter, but I quickly wanted to share with you how exactly you make quinoa, buckwheat and brown rice so that you can master every recipe in the rest of the book. The trick to making them all delicious is adding a few ingredients to the water when you put the grain in at the beginning, so that it absorbs all the flavour. I use lemon, tamari and salt to do this.

QUINOA

Serves 1

⅓ mug quinoa (90g)

juice of 1 lime or lemon

1 teaspoon tamari

sprinkling of salt – I like using my herb or chilli salt (recipe on page 19)

Place the quinoa in a sieve and rinse with cold water until the water that comes through is totally clear.

Place the quinoa in a saucepan with 1 mug (300ml) boiling water. Stir the lemon juice in with the tamari and salt.

Let the quinoa boil for a minute or two, then let it simmer for another 10–15 minutes, covered, until all the water has been evaporated and the quinoa is fluffy, but not mushy.

Allow the quinoa to cool before placing it in an airtight container, then store in the fridge for up to a week.

BUCKWHEAT

Serves 1

⅓ mug buckwheat (65g)

juice of 1 lime or lemon

1 teaspoon tamari

sprinkling of salt – I like using my herb or chilli salt (recipe on page 19)

Place the buckwheat in a sieve and rinse with cold water until the water that comes through is totally clear.

Place the buckwheat in a saucepan with 1 mug (300ml) boiling water. Stir the lemon juice in with the tamari and salt.

Let the buckwheat boil for a minute or two, then let it simmer for another 10–15 minutes, until all the water has been evaporated and the buckwheat is ever so slightly hard and nutty, but not crunchy or soggy.

Allow the buckwheat to cool before placing it in an airtight container, then store in the fridge for up to a week.

BROWN RICE

Serves 1

⅓ mug brown rice (90g)

juice of 1 lime or lemon

1 teaspoon tamari

sprinkling of salt – I like using my herb or chilli
    salt (recipe on page 19)

1 tablespoon olive oil

Place the rice in a saucepan with 1½ mugs
(450ml) water, the lime or lemon juice, tamari
and salt.

Bring the pan to the boil and let it bubble for 5
minutes or so, then simmer for about 45 minutes,
covered, until the rice is soft, but not soggy, and
all the water has evaporated. You'll need to stir the
rice and may need to add more boiling water as it
cooks – make sure the rice never runs out of water
until it is done.

Once it's finished cooking and there's no water
left in the pan, stir in the olive oil – this adds a
delicious flavour and stops the rice from getting
sticky.

Allow the rice to cool before placing it in an
airtight container, then store in the fridge for up
to a week.

Top tip

For the last couple of minutes of cooking your
grains, turn the heat off and allow the last little bit
of water to evaporate without the heat. This means
that the grains won't stick to the bottom of your
pan and burn it.

EASY VEGGIE STOCK

I know that veggie stock doesn't sound overly
exciting, but it's an amazing thing to keep in the
freezer as it automatically adds so much flavour to
whatever you're cooking. Plus, it's a great way to
use up old veggies! I love cooking my grains in it
or using it instead of water in cooking.

makes 1 litre

2 carrots, roughly chopped

2 onions, quartered

2 tomatoes, quartered

2 stalks of celery, roughly chopped

2 cloves of garlic, peeled

2 bay leaves

6 peppercorns

Add all the vegetables and garlic to a large
saucepan along with the bay leaves and
peppercorns.

Fill the pan about a third full with water and
bring it to the boil, then allow it to simmer for
about 20 minutes.

Once it's cooked, drain it through a colander
into another saucepan and collect the liquid.
Discard the veggies.

Either use the stock within 3 days or freeze it.

Top tip

Make this in big batches and then store it in
freezer bags in the freezer so that you've always got
some lying around.

COOK'S NOTES: MUGS

When I first started cooking, my main priority was that each meal would be quick and easy to make, so I
didn't even think about buying scales and measuring ingredients. Instead, I simply measured everything
with a standard-sized coffee mug. When I started the blog all my recipes were in mugs and it's how I
always work, so I've included the mug measurements in every recipe so that you can cook in the same way
if you like. If not, then I've also included the grams and millilitre measurements for everything.

GRAINS

a very good place to start

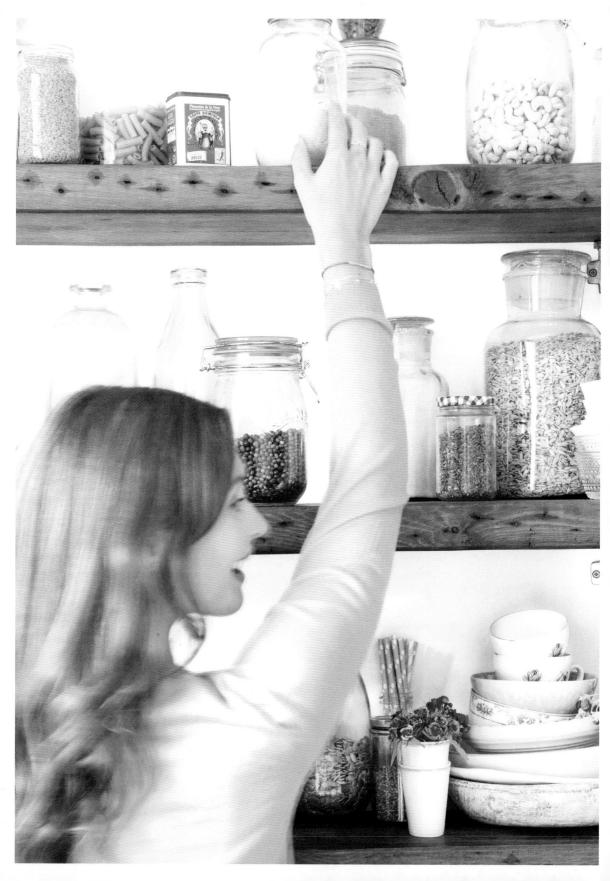

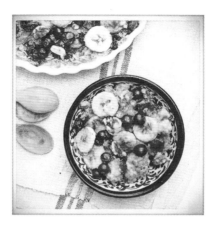

grains

I love whole grains; they form a huge part of my diet and make up the basis of most of my meals. If you're eating a plant-based diet, they're a really important source of goodness as they're full of vitamins, minerals, fibre and protein – all of which you need to look and feel awesome. They're also so versatile and work in absolutely everything, you can eat them warm or cold, mixing them into everything from stews and soups to salads and risottos.

All the grains I eat are gluten free, so I don't eat things like bulgur wheat or couscous. Instead, my savoury staples are brown rice, buckwheat and quinoa, all of which are really versatile and taste delicious when cooked in the right way. The other grain I'm obsessed with is oats, mainly because porridge is one of my favourite foods, but also because they're amazing in baking and granola making.

I have to quickly mention that quinoa and buckwheat are actually pseudo-grains as they're technically seeds, but we eat them in the same way that we eat grains, so like brown rice, they seem to fit better in this chapter than they do alongside

the almonds and pumpkin seeds! The awesome thing about all four of these grains is that not only are they really good for you, they're really inexpensive, so you can make them the basis of your meal very easily and then add seasonal veggies or fruits to them and you get something delicious and nutritious without a big price tag.

I buy these grains in bulk so that I always have them to hand, and then store them in glass jars, although any airtight container is perfect. They need to live at room temperature when they're raw and then once they've been cooked, they should be stored in the fridge. You can make large quantities of these grains and then store the leftovers in the freezer so that there's always something delicious waiting for you after a busy day.

The thing about grains is that they often get a bad reputation and people tend to avoid them as part of the carbohydrate fear, but if you eat the right ones, they're pretty incredible. They're an amazing source of energy, great for keeping your mood balanced and also an important food if you're trying to lose weight as they're filling, but nutritious. I'll go into more detail about the individual benefits of each grain later on, but for now I just wanted to say, please don't be scared of them!

I know that grains are sometimes considered to be quite bland, so it's really important to master the art of cooking them in a way that automatically gives them flavour. The trick is to add a mixture of ingredients to the water as soon as you put the grain into the pan, so as the grain expands and absorbs the water, it also absorbs the flavours of whatever you've added. Doing this makes a huge difference to the final taste as the flavours are absorbed right into the middle of the grain, much more so than if you added the same ingredients right at the end. I do this trick with all of them, even the oats when I make porridge. It's really the simplest trick, but it does absolute wonders.

With oats, I add things like berries, sliced banana, honey, coconut oil, cinnamon and almond butter to the water or milk at the beginning so that each bite is so deliciously rich and sweet. With rice, buckwheat and quinoa, I add more savoury ingredients, normally a mixture of lime, lemon or apple cider vinegar, plus some tamari or miso paste, dried herbs, salt and pepper. You can then add anything you like at the end, including more of these ingredients, but you'll just be building up from a more flavoursome base so it's easier to create absolutely delicious dishes.

Each grain is really different though and each has its own awesome advantages, which I've outlined below so you can become really familiar with them all and know which is best when!

QUINOA

Quinoa has been having a bit of a moment over the last few years, which is fantastic as more and more people are discovering how amazing it tastes and how good it makes you feel. It's an ancient grain though and was probably first cultivated about five thousand years ago. It originally comes from the Andes in Bolivia, where it was an essential part of the Inca diet. It comes in a few different varieties too: white quinoa, red quinoa and black quinoa, and you can also buy quinoa flour. Quinoa flour is pretty savoury, so it's not ideal in sweet baking, but it's great in everything else.

I absolutely adore the white, red and black quinoa grains and use them all the time. The three have quite distinct differences in taste and texture. White quinoa has the most subtle flavour and a lighter, fluffier texture, whereas black quinoa is much nuttier and has a denser texture, and red quinoa sits somewhere between the two. I tend to use either white quinoa on its own or a mix of the three, with the ratio being about two thirds white quinoa to one third red and black. Don't worry though as although white quinoa is white, it's not refined, it's just naturally much lighter (although I'd say the colour was actually more beige, like brown rice, rather than pure white).

One of the best things about quinoa is that it's so nutrient-dense. It's a complete protein source, which is quite rare in plant-based foods. This, coupled with its high fibre content, means that it works really well to regulate your blood sugar, which is vital to prevent and reverse illness. It's also very anti-inflammatory and contains an amazing array of vitamins and minerals, including iron, magnesium, manganese and calcium. These are all essential for healthy bones and muscles as well as energy metabolism and production.

The other brilliant thing about quinoa is that it's very quick to make. It takes just over ten minutes to go from packet to plate, so it's great if you're in a hurry. All you have to do is pour it out of its packet into your pan, add boiling water, herbs and lemon and then let it boil for about ten minutes. You don't have to wash it or soak it like pulses. Quinoa grains are smaller and lighter than both buckwheat and brown rice, so it's best served as the main dish with veggies on the side, rather than as a side to things like curries or stews or used in risottos, as it easily gets lost in those situations. My favourite way to eat it is simply with lots of sautéed veggies and a dressing of tamari, tahini and lemon – so simple, yet so good (page 36).

Quinoa is pretty easy to get hold of and you can find it in almost all supermarkets now, including Sainsbury's and Tesco. Of course you can also buy it online or from any health-food shop.

BUCKWHEAT

Like quinoa, buckwheat is an ancient grain that has been cultivated since about 4000 BC. It originates in Eastern Europe and Asia and comes from the seed of a fruit related to rhubarb. Despite being so old, so delicious and so nutritious, it's a pretty underrated food in most of the Western world. It doesn't get half the attention that quinoa does and you very rarely see it on a menu, even at health-food restaurants. I have a feeling that it will have a quinoa moment soon though as it's really delicious, but for now it can be our secret to enjoy!

In terms of goodness, it's pretty similar to quinoa as it's full of plant protein, fibre, vitamins and minerals. It's an amazing food for balancing blood sugar and works wonders for your energy levels as its high level of fibre means it's broken down and released into the bloodstream slowly over several hours. It also contains lots of iron and magnesium, both of which are important for beautiful, glowing skin.

Buckwheat (also known as buckwheat groats) is the perfect cross between quinoa and brown rice; it's denser and nuttier than quinoa, but not as substantial as rice. This means that unlike quinoa, it works really well as the side dish to curries and stews as it stands out on its own. The groats also work incredibly well in risottos instead of rice. I love making risottos by roasting root veggies and

then puréeing them with things like coconut milk and lemon juice, before stirring the creamy purée into the buckwheat – honestly, the most delicious thing ever! You can totally use brown rice for this, but it's nice to make a change from rice and buckwheat is much quicker to make. Like quinoa, buckwheat only takes about ten minutes to cook, so it's very easy to prepare.

You can also get buckwheat flour, which I use all the time. It's pretty interchangeable with brown rice flour and both have the same effect in baking. They're my favourite gluten-free flours to bake with, so you'll find loads of recipes using them throughout the book.

The other type of buckwheat you can get is sprouted buckwheat. This is when the buckwheat groats have been soaked and dehydrated, causing them to be super crunchy (this is different to roasted buckwheat or kasha). Sprouted buckwheat is an incredible addition to granola and tastes amazing as a topping for smoothie bowls as it's amazingly crispy. You can't cook it though. I got confused once when I first starting cooking with buckwheat and not knowing the difference between raw sprouted buckwheat and normal buckwheat, I tried to boil the sprouts. Needless to say it was a total disaster and they turned into a soggy mess – do not try this at home!

Buckwheat is harder to find than quinoa as it's not available in mainstream supermarkets yet, but it is easy to buy online from places like Planet Organic or even Amazon. It's also sold in all health-food shops.

BROWN RICE

In some ways brown rice is probably the least exciting of all the grains I'm talking about, as it's not new and exotic like quinoa and buckwheat. This doesn't, however, mean that it's not awesome – it really is! I know people eat a lot of rice, but it always seems to be white. This really confuses me and I just can't get my head around why people eat white rice over brown rice, not just because white rice isn't really great for us and brown rice is super nutritious, but because white rice also tastes of nothing and brown rice is delicious.

Both brown and white rice come from the same grain, but the difference between them is the process by which they're made. To make brown rice only the outermost layer of the grain is removed, which means that almost all of the goodness is retained. Whereas to make white rice, the rice has to be milled to remove another couple of layers and then polished, which means that almost all the goodness is taken away. Between sixty and eighty per cent of the vitamins are removed, plus almost all the dietary fibre and essential fatty acids. So brown rice is full of goodness, whereas white rice is refined and lacking in almost everything! Each grain of brown rice is packed with B vitamins, which are essential for energy, as well as manganese, selenium, magnesium and iron.

Brown rice also has a richer flavour and, like buckwheat, it's still nutty. My favourite way to eat brown rice is to cook it and then once all the water has been absorbed, I add some tomato purée, some miso paste, a little garlic and some black beans. I eat this with a mashed avocado and it's beyond delicious – the best five-minute meal ever. Brown rice goes with basically everything though, from risottos (page 54) to sides for curries and chillies to salads. Of course you can spice it up by using more exotic wild rice, which is totally delicious, but it's not as easy to find and it is more expensive, so brown rice is my staple.

OATS

Oats are probably my favourite of all the grains we're talking about because they're naturally really sweet and I have a serious sweet tooth! Honestly, I sometimes dream of steaming hot bowls of Creamy Coconut Porridge (page 57) topped with fresh berries, cacao nibs, raisins, toasted almonds, banana slices and honey. I know that's quite sad, but I just love good food and when it's made right, porridge is just heavenly. Of course there is so much more you can do with oats than just porridge, and even with porridge itself there are so many variations, from a classic banana and cinnamon to carrot cake porridge, coconut porridge, chocolate porridge and one of my all-time favourites, Apple and Cinnamon Porridge Bake (page 58).

You can also use your oats to make sweet, creamy Oat Milk (page 20) or mix them with nuts and seeds to make home-made Cinnamon Pecan Granola (page 76) or muesli, bake them as Flapjacks (page 63) or Simple Oat Cookies (page 62), blend them into smoothies and even grind them up to make flour. They're amazingly versatile things and their sweet flavour and crumbly texture really adds to almost any dish. Plus oats are incredible for us, especially as their fibre content is so high, so they really help to balance blood sugar and keep you energised for hours, which is why they make such a great breakfast. The other awesome thing about oats is that they're really cheap, so you can make things like porridge for breakfast without spending a lot. You can use oat milk and water, oats, bananas and raisins to create something delicious and easy without breaking the bank.

There's always some confusion as to whether oats are gluten-free and the answer is that, by and large, unless you have a very severe allergy to gluten, then oats are amazing. They don't actually contain gluten, but they're normally handled in factories that do and therefore cannot be labelled 'certified gluten-free' in case of any potential cross-contamination. I'm not a coeliac, but I do have a pretty serious intolerance to gluten in the sense that it causes my lymph nodes to swell and ache, makes my tummy swell like crazy until I look pregnant, I feel like I've been poisoned and my torso goes burning hot, but none of these things happen to me when I eat oats. If you are coeliac, then you can buy gluten-free oats. They're much more expensive, but they are handled in factories that are certified gluten-free so you're totally safe.

There are lots of different types of oats around: steel-cut oats, rolled oats, old-fashioned oats, quick oats and porridge oats, and it gets pretty confusing trying to work out what the difference is between them all! The short answer is that the differences aren't huge and you can use any of them in any of these recipes. The time you'll notice a difference is in your porridge as the texture does vary a little. Steel-cut oats are where the oat groat is split into several pieces. They take slightly longer to cook and retain their original texture better than rolled oats, which are steamed and then pressed between rollers and dried. This means that rolled oats cook quicker and are a little softer. Porridge oats can be either steel-cut or rolled oats. And just to make it more confusing, old-fashioned oats are the same as rolled oats, just with a different name! Quick oats are oats that have been pressed a little thinner than rolled oats, so they cook quicker but retain less of their texture. These are my least favourite of all the different varieties and I tend to avoid them.

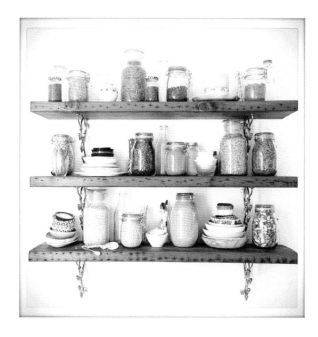

EASY QUINOA *with Sautéed Veggies*

This was the first quinoa dish I ever made and I still come back to it time and time again. It's very simple, but it's always such a hit and everyone loves it. The tamari, tahini and lemon make the quinoa amazingly flavoursome, while the broccoli and courgettes add lot of green goodness. It tastes incredible with a side of cinnamon and paprika-roasted Sweet Potato Wedges (page 132) or with a generous dollop of creamy, home-made Hummus (page 102).

Serves 2

⅔ mug quinoa (180g)
juice of 1 lemon
3 tablespoons tamari
2 courgettes
1 small broccoli
olive oil
1 tablespoon tahini
salt and pepper

Place the quinoa in a sieve and rinse with cold water until the water that comes through is totally clear.

Place the quinoa in a saucepan with 2 mugs (600ml) boiling water, the juice of the lemon and a tablespoon of tamari.

Let the quinoa boil for a minute or two, then let it simmer for another 10–15 minutes, covered, until all the water has been evaporated and the quinoa is fluffy, but not mushy.

While the quinoa cooks, slice the courgettes in half and then chop them into thin half-moons. Once you've done that, cut the broccoli into small florets.

Place the courgette slices and broccoli florets into a frying pan with some olive oil, another tablespoon of tamari, salt and pepper and allow them to cook for 5–7 minutes.

Once the quinoa has cooked and there is no water in the pan, stir the tahini in and the final tablespoon of tamari before mixing it all with the sautéed veggies and a drizzling of olive oil.

Top tip

Make this as an on-the-go work lunch. It stores well in the fridge for a few days and tastes equally delicious cold – just add a drizzle of olive oil and a sprinkling of pepper when you're ready to eat it.

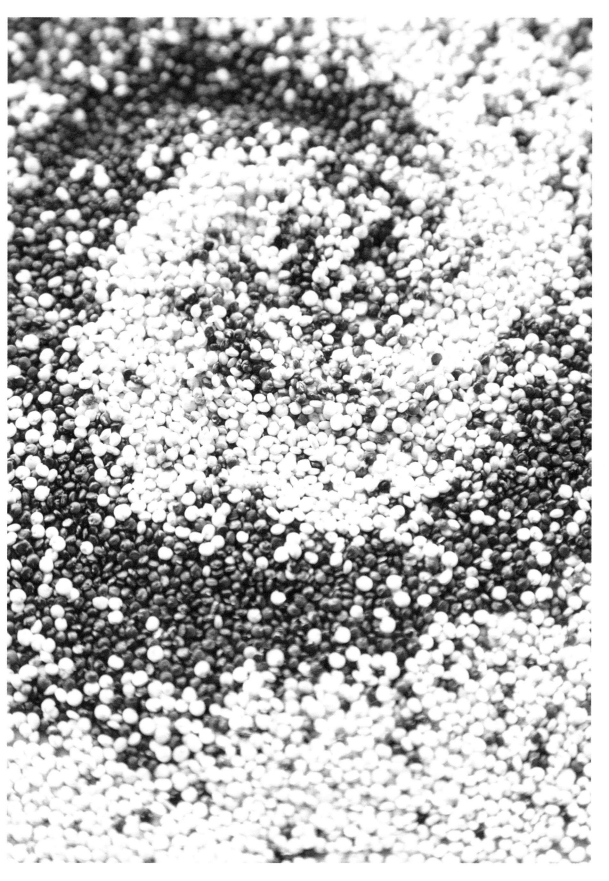

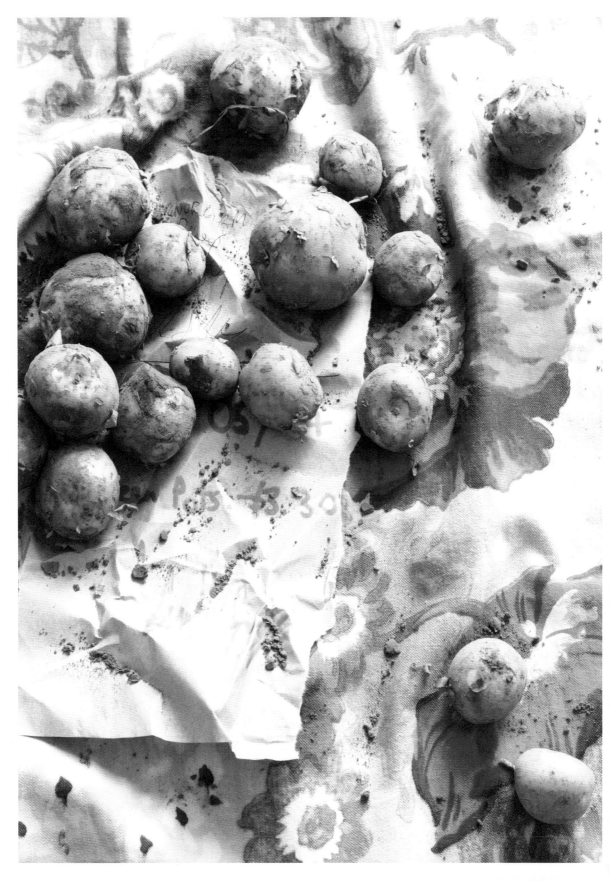

GNOCCHI WITH PEA PESTO

Before I changed my diet, gnocchi was always my go-to meal at an Italian restaurant. It took me a while to figure out how to make it healthy, but I think I really have done it here! I have to warn you that the colour isn't as beautiful as brown rice flour isn't as white as the flour you normally use, but once you've mixed it with lots of pesto, you won't realise. Nutritional yeast is a deactivated strain of yeast. It has a cheese-like flavour, which is why I add it to my pesto, but if you don't have any then don't worry, it's not essential. Please don't use baker's yeast as a substitute, it's completely different!

Serves 4

For the pesto

1 mug peas (150g)
60g fresh basil
1 mug brazil nuts (120g)
10 tablespoons olive oil
2 teaspoons nutritional yeast

For the gnocchi

8 potatoes (1kg)
3 tablespoons apple purée
   (recipe on page 19)
2 mugs buckwheat/brown rice
   flour (400g)
salt and pepper

For the pesto

Place the peas in a saucepan with enough cold water to cover and allow them to heat up until they're boiling. Then drain them and place a food processor.

Tear off the basil leaves and blend them in the processor along with the brazil nuts, olive oil, 4 tablespoons water and the nutritional yeast, until smooth and creamy.

For the gnocchi

Place the potatoes in a large saucepan and cover them with cold water. Allow them to boil for about 30 minutes, until they're nicely tender.

Drain the potatoes and then allow them to cool for a few minutes before peeling their skins off.

Next, mash the potatoes with the apple purée, salt and pepper until they are totally smooth.

Once the potatoes are smooth, stir in the buckwheat or brown rice flour.

Spread flour over the work surface and roll the gnocchi mix out over it, separating the mix into six long, sausage-shaped rolls. Cut the rolls into small pieces.

Finally, fill a large saucepan with boiling water, add a little salt and then drop the gnocchi in. After a couple of minutes the gnocchi should rise to the top.

Drain the gnocchi and place it back into the pan with the pesto. Heat for a couple of minutes until the pesto is warm and then serve.

WARM WILD RICE SALAD

This salad makes rice more delicious then ever. Cooking it with garlic and tamari gives it such a rich, beautiful flavour that goes so well with the crunchy pine nuts and sweet, juicy raisins. It's a great side dish for almost anything. I love it served with my steamed Broccoli with a Tahini Dressing (page 159) and some home-made Classic Guacamole (page 32), although it tastes amazing on its own too.

Serves 4

1 mug black or red rice (I prefer black rice, but red rice is
    perfect too) (300g)
3 cloves of garlic, peeled and crushed
2 tablespoons tamari
1 mug raisins (200g)
¾ mug pine nuts (100g)
1 tablespoon tahini
juice of 1 lemon
olive oil
salt and pepper

Place the rice in a large saucepan, covering it with boiling water. As the rice begins to boil, add the garlic and the tamari.

Allow the pan to simmer for about 45 minutes, during which time you will need to add more boiling water to ensure that it never goes dry.

While the rice cooks, soak the raisins in a bowl of boiling water – this makes them softer and juicier.

Just before the rice finishes cooking, place the pine nuts in a frying pan and toast them. This should take just a minute or so and doesn't require any oil as they'll release their own. You want them to be golden brown but not burnt.

Finally, once the rice is cooked and all the water has been evaporated, drain the raisins and stir them into the pan alongside the toasted pine nuts, tahini, lemon juice, salt and pepper and a generous drizzle of olive oil.

Top tip

This is another great meal to take on the go with you as whilst I like to serve it warm, it also tastes amazing cold and lasts about a week in the fridge.

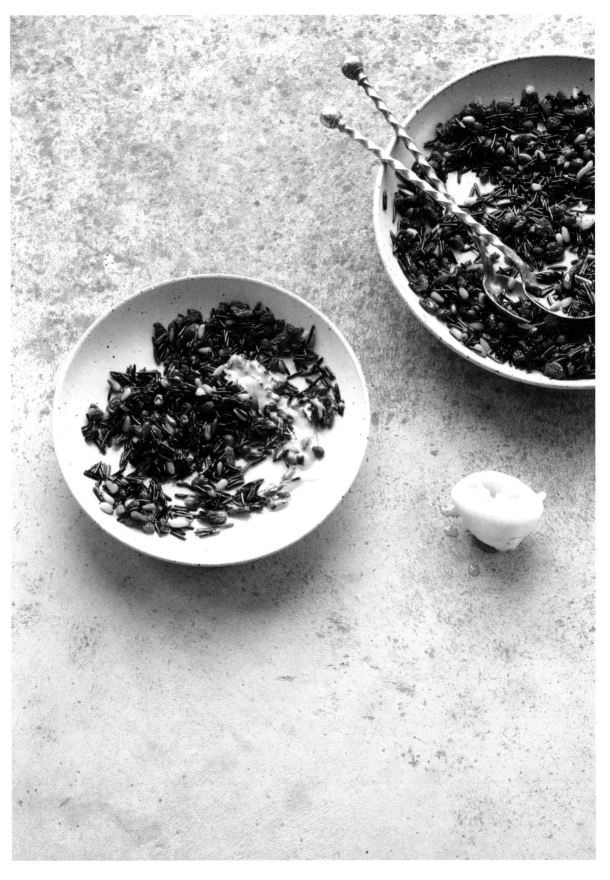

BUCKWHEAT AND BEETROOT RISOTTO

I taught this recipe at my cooking classes last year and it was such a hit. It's a really surprising dish as it's so simple, but tastes so amazing, and it's the most beautiful, vibrant pink colour, which makes it look so delicious! It's a warming dish too – perfect healthy comfort food. The puréed beetroot coupled with the coconut milk really makes the dish so creamy, while the lemon adds a gentle tanginess that enhances all the other flavours.

Serves 4
5-6 beetroots (1.5kg)
2 mugs buckwheat (400g)
juice of 1 lemon
1 x 400ml tin coconut milk
salt and pepper

Start by roasting the beetroots whole, with their skins on, in a 210°C (fan 190°C) oven. They will take about an hour to cook. You don't need to add any olive oil.

Once the beetroots are nice and soft and the skin is becoming crispy, take the beetroots out of the oven and leave them to cool for a minute.

Place the buckwheat in a sieve and rinse with cold water until the water that comes through is totally clear.

Place the buckwheat in a saucepan with 3½ mugs (1 litre) boiling water.

Let the buckwheat boil for a minute or two, then let it simmer for another 10–15 minutes, until all the water has been evaporated and the buckwheat is ever so slightly hard and nutty, but not crunchy or soggy.

Peel the skin off the beetroots – it should come off easily with a knife and fork. Place the flesh into a food processor with the lemon juice, coconut milk, salt and pepper and blend. The mixture should come out smooth.

Once the buckwheat has cooked, stir in the beetroot, heat through and then serve.

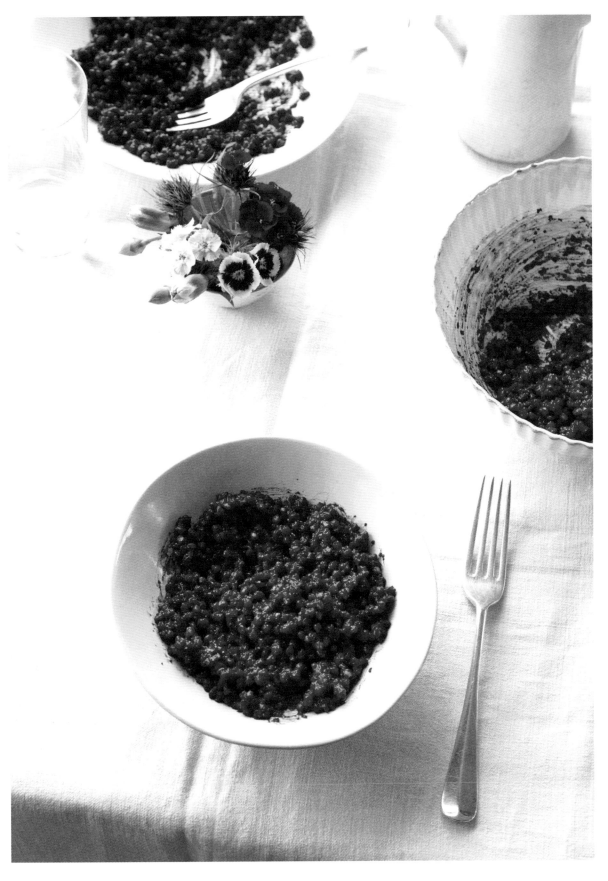

CREAMY POLENTA *with mushrooms and Crispy Kale*

Polenta is an Italian staple. It's made from ground corn, which you then cook with water until it becomes thick and creamy. It's amazing comfort food as it's so warming and nourishing. I love it served with crispy roasted kale and sautéed mushrooms infused with tamari and fresh thyme. It's amazing with a side of Sweet Potato Wedges (page 132) too.

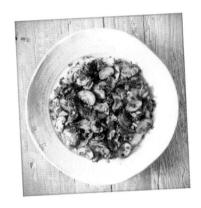

Serves 4

⅔ mug polenta (150g)
250g kale
500g button mushrooms
2 tablespoons tamari (soy sauce will
   also work)
dozen sprigs of fresh thyme
olive oil
juice of ½ lemon
salt and pepper

Preheat the oven to 190°C (fan 170°C).

Pour 1 litre water into a large saucepan with a lid and bring it to the boil.

Once it's boiling, turn down the heat and then gradually pour in the polenta, stirring it continuously as it's poured in.

Once the polenta is in the pan, keep stirring for a couple of minutes until it's nice and thick.

At this point, place the lid on the pan and every 5 minutes, stir it again – just like making risotto.

Tear the kale off its stems and place it in a baking tray with a little olive oil and salt. Bake the kale for about 20 minutes until it's nice and crispy.

Next, slice the mushrooms into thin pieces and place them in a frying pan with the tamari and the leaves of the thyme and sauté for 5–10 minutes.

Once everything has finished cooking, stir the lemon juice into the polenta before pouring the polenta into bowls.

Drizzle a little olive oil over the bowls and then add the crispy kale and sautéed mushrooms on top.

QUINOA PIZZA CRUST

This is the simplest pizza crust; it requires so few ingredients and no complicated cooking, which is always good! It's been a favourite on my blog for a while and everyone just loves it, which is why I decided that it had to go in the book too. You can add any topping to it – I love using a tomato purée or pesto base and then piling it high with fresh veggies, from artichoke hearts to rocket, cherry tomatoes, mushrooms and sweetcorn.

makes a 20cm pizza

For the base
¾ mug quinoa (195g)
1 teaspoon apple cider vinegar
2 teaspoons dried mixed herbs (I used herbes de Provence and oregano)
sprinkling of chilli flakes
olive oil, for greasing
salt

For the toppings
2 tablespoons tomato purée
12 cherry tomatoes
handful of pitted black olives
2-3 tablespoons artichokes from a jar
handful of rocket

For the base
Soak the quinoa overnight or for about 8 hours in cold water. The best way to do this is to put the quinoa in a large bowl and cover it with water, making sure that it's covered by a few centimetres. Then leave this to one side.

Once you're ready to make the pizza, preheat the oven to 210°C (fan 190°C).

Drain any water left in the quinoa bowl, before putting the quinoa into a food processor with the apple cider vinegar, herbs, chilli flakes and salt. Blend for a few minutes until a smooth dough forms – it should look a bit like a pancake mix.

Line the bottom of a 20cm pizza pan or cake pan with olive oil and pour the mix in, then bake for about 15–20 minutes, until the base is firm – it cooks pretty quickly though.

For the toppings
Remove and add your toppings. Either place the pizza back in the oven for a few minutes to warm them or enjoy your toppings raw!

QUINOA TABBOULEH

Tabbouleh is a delicious Middle Eastern dish, which is traditionally made with bulgur wheat. Sadly, bulgur wheat isn't gluten-free, so I like to use quinoa instead – although the same recipe is also delicious with buckwheat. The whole dish tastes incredibly light and fresh thanks to the fresh coriander and lemon juice, while the tahini adds a rich flavour and a little creaminess to each bite. I love this served with a simple rocket salad, my Spicy Roasted Chickpeas (page 112) and some Falafels (page 107).

Serves 4
1½ mugs quinoa (390g)
200g fresh coriander
8 tomatoes
¾ mug pine nuts (100g)
2 tablespoons tahini
4 tablespoons olive oil
juice of 2 lemons
salt and pepper

Place the quinoa in a sieve and rinse with cold water until the water that comes through is totally clear.

Place the quinoa in a saucepan with 3 mugs (900ml) boiling water. Let the quinoa boil for a minute or two, then let it simmer for another 10–15 minutes, covered, until all the water has been evaporated and the quinoa is fluffy, but not mushy.

While the quinoa cooks, finely chop the coriander leaves (I find it easiest to do this by placing the leaves in a mug and chopping them with a pair of scissors). Chop the tomatoes into small, salsa-like squares.

Toast the pine nuts in a dry frying pan – this should take just a couple of minutes.

Once the quinoa has finished cooking, allow it to cool.

Mix in the coriander, chopped tomato, tahini, olive oil, lemon juice and toasted pine nuts before sprinkling it all with salt and pepper.

Top tip
This is a great picnic dish as it's easy to make, is meant to be served cold and goes with everything!

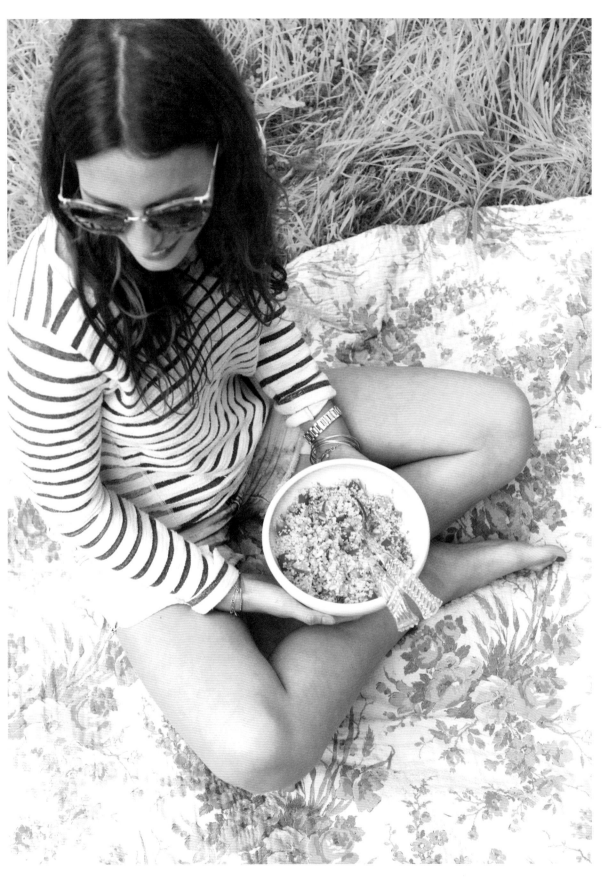

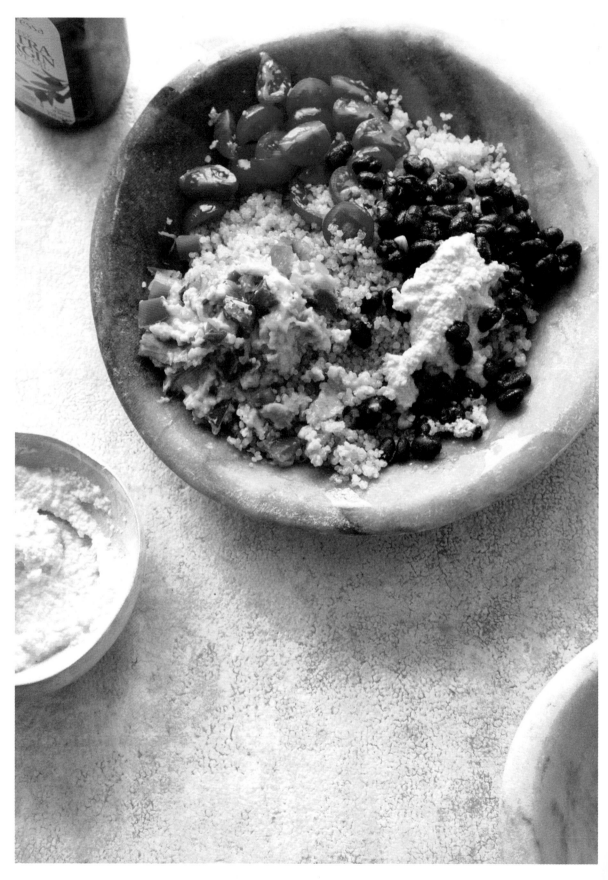

MEXICAN QUINOA BOWL

This is one of my favourite recipes in the book – it's so incredibly delicious and I have to admit that I often get cravings for it! It is super quick and easy to make while the quinoa is cooking you can get started on making the mountains of fresh guacamole, creamy cashew cheese, tomato salsa and garlicky black beans. You will love the amazing mix of intense flavours!

Serves 4

For the cashew cream

2 mugs cashew nuts (400g)
juice of 1 lemon
1 tablespoon tamari
salt and pepper

For the quinoa

1 mug quinoa (260g)
juice of 1 lemon
salt and pepper

For the guacamole

4 avocados
6 tomatoes, chopped into tiny
    pieces
1 jalapeño pepper, deseeded and
    chopped into tiny pieces
handful of fresh coriander,
    finely chopped
juice of 3 limes
salt and pepper

For the salsa

3 tomatoes
juice of 1 lime
3 tablespoons olive oil
salt and pepper

For the black beans

2 x 400g tins black beans
3 cloves of garlic, peeled and
    crushed
olive oil
salt

For the cashew cream

Soak the cashews in a bowl of cold water for 4 hours.

Drain the water that the cashew nuts have been soaking in. Blend the nuts in a food processor with the juice of the lemon, tamari, ½ mug (150ml) fresh water, salt and pepper, until smooth and creamy. This may take a couple of minutes.

For the quinoa

Place the quinoa in a sieve and rinse with cold water until the water that comes through is totally clear.

Place the quinoa in a saucepan with 2 mugs (600ml) boiling water and a little salt, pepper and lemon juice.

Let the quinoa boil for a minute or two, then simmer for another 10–15 minutes, covered, until all the water has been evaporated and the quinoa is fluffy.

For the guacamole

Cut the avocados in half and scoop out their flesh, placing it into a bowl. Use a fork to mash the avocados. Stir the tomato, jalapeño pepper and the coriander into the mashed avocado with the lime juice, salt and pepper.

For the salsa

Slice the tomatoes into quarters, then finely chop these into small squares. Place the tomatoes in a bowl, pour over the lime juice and olive oil and add a little salt and pepper.

For the black beans

Drain the black beans, then pour them into a large saucepan. Add the garlic to the pan, along with a drizzle of olive oil and some salt. Heat through for a few minutes.

To serve, place the quinoa in the middle of the bowl, then add the cashew cream, black beans, salsa and guacamole around the quinoa.

QUINOA AND TURMERIC FRITTERS

Turmeric is one of the most healing foods on the planet as it's so incredibly anti-inflammatory and as a result, it's long been a celebrated spice in Chinese and Indian medicine. It has a warm, peppery flavour that works so well in this dish to add a deep flavour to the quinoa fritters. I love these served either over a bed of rocket or sautéed spinach with a side of the tomatoes from my Pan con Tomate recipe (page 135) or the cashew cream from my Mexican Quinoa Bowl recipe (page 49).

Serves 6

1 large sweet potato (340g)
1 mug quinoa (260g)
2 lemons
4 tablespoons almond butter
   (recipe on page 24)
4 tablespoons tomato purée
8 tablespoons buckwheat or
   brown rice flour
2 teaspoons ground turmeric
2 teaspoons ground cumin
olive oil
salt and pepper

Top tip

If you have a nut allergy, swap the almond butter for tahini.

Start by peeling the sweet potato, then chop it into small pieces and either steam or boil them for about 20 minutes, until they're really soft.

While they cook, rinse the quinoa with cold water until the water runs totally clear.

Place the quinoa in a saucepan with the juice from one of the lemons and 2 mugs (600ml) boiling water. Boil for a minute or two, then let it simmer for another 10–15 minutes, covered, until all the water has been evaporated and the quinoa is fluffy.

Drain the sweet potatoes once they are soft and blend them in a food processor with the juice of the other lemon plus the almond butter, tomato purée, flour, turmeric, cumin, salt and pepper until totally smooth.

Preheat the oven to 200°C (fan 180°C).

Place the sweet potato mix into a large mixing bowl and stir in the cooked quinoa (ensuring that there's no water left in the quinoa pan) until nice and sticky.

Grease a large baking tray with olive oil and scoop 2 tablespoons worth of the mix onto it to make a circle, then do the rest with the remaining mix so that you have twelve circular fritters.

Bake for 20 minutes, until the fritters are perfectly stuck together.

You can then eat them like this or place them in a frying pan with a little olive oil and fry each side for a couple of minutes so that they're a bit crispy.

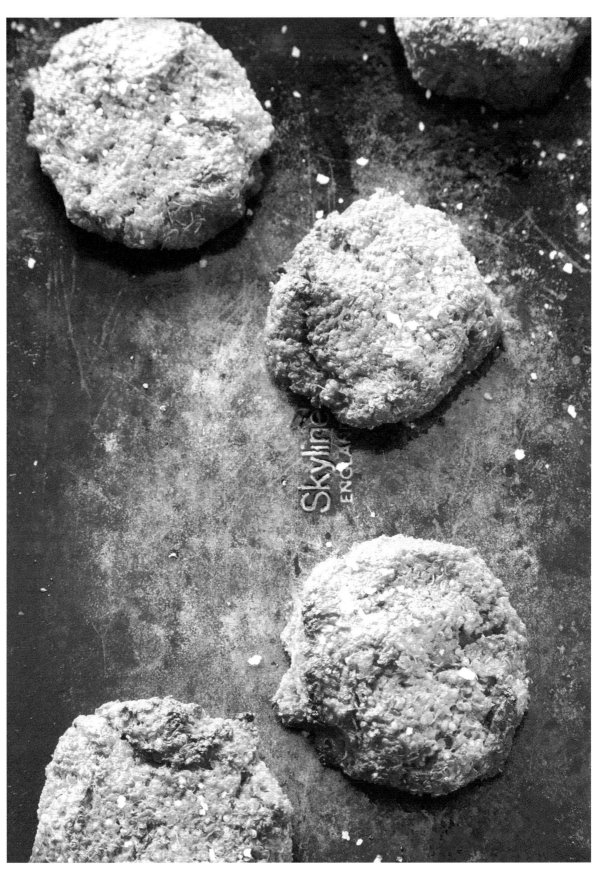

BUCKWHEAT FOCACCIA

This Buckwheat Focaccia is the perfect accompaniment to any meal. It tastes amazing dunked into soups or used as a base for guacamole, salsa or hummus. It's also a delicious addition to a salad and works really well if you're taking food on the go. It's a very simple recipe too and only takes 5 minutes to put together before you bake it, which is always great.

Makes 1 loaf

½ mug olive oil (150ml)
2 tablespoons chia seeds
3 tablespoons apple cider vinegar
2½ mugs buckwheat flour (500g)
1 mug sun-dried tomatoes (180g)
1 mug pitted olives (180g)
20g fresh rosemary sprigs
coconut oil, for greasing
salt and pepper

Preheat the oven to 200°C (fan 180°C).

Simply place 1½ mugs (450ml) water, the olive oil, chia seeds, apple cider vinegar, buckwheat flour and lots of salt and pepper in a mixing bowl.

Whisk it all together until the mix is smooth.

Stir in the sun-dried tomatoes and olives. Tear the leaves off half of the rosemary and mix them in.

Grease a baking dish with coconut oil, then pour in the focaccia mix and layer the other half of the rosemary sprigs on the top.

Place the dish in the oven and bake for about 30 minutes, until the top starts to turn a golden brown.

Top tip

Try brushing a layer of olive oil over the top of the focaccia midway through baking to give a beautiful golden glow.

FRESH SPRING ROLLS

These fresh spring rolls make for the perfect appetiser or light lunch. Every bite just tastes so fresh and nutritious, while the mango dipping sauce adds such a beautifully creamy element, as well as a sweet flavour that really complements the raw veggies in the rolls. These are incredibly portable too and they store well, so you can make them the night before and then take them to work with you for lunch.

makes 16 rolls

For the dip

2 ripe mangoes
I ripe avocado
juice of I lime
2 tablespoons olive oil
2 tablespoons tahini
I teaspoon chilli flakes
large handful of fresh coriander
4cm piece of fresh ginger

For the rolls

I ripe mango
16 rice paper wraps
3 carrots, thinly sliced
2 red peppers, thinly sliced
I large cucumber, thinly sliced
juice of 2 limes
salt and pepper

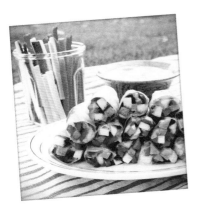

For the dip

Peel the mangos using a vegetable peeler and cut their flesh from the stone, then place the flesh into a blender.

Add the avocado flesh, lime juice, olive oil, tahini and chilli flakes to the blender with a little salt.

Cut the coriander leaves from the stalks and peel the ginger and slice it into a few pieces before adding them both to the blender too.

Blend until smooth and creamy.

For the rolls

Peel the mango using a vegetable peeler and cut its flesh from the stone, then chop into thin slices.

Once you've done that, prepare the rice paper wraps. Simply dip them in hot water for about 10 seconds to soften before placing them flat on a chopping board to dry for a couple of minutes.

Once the wraps are dry, place a heaped teaspoon of the dip along the middle of each one, then place a selection of the sliced mango and veggies in the middle and squeeze a few drops of lime juice over them, plus a little salt and pepper.

Wrap them up and dunk them into the dip!

Top tip

If you don't have any rice paper wraps, then try making these in nori sheets instead – they're delicious!

BUTTERNUT SQUASH RISOTTO

This healthy take on a classic risotto is another favourite recipe from the blog. It's just as creamy and delicious as a classic risotto, but it contains much more beautifying goodness. The brown rice tastes just as great as white, but it also adds in so much fibre, as well as an amazing array of vitamins and minerals. The beauty of the dish though is the creamy purée made with roasted squash cubes infused with paprika and cumin, a little tahini, apple cider vinegar and nutritional yeast. This is stirred into the rice and then topped with extra bites of soft squash and a sprinkling of coriander. Try adding steamed asparagus and broccoli on top of your risotto bowl for extra goodness.

Serves 4

¾ mug brown rice (200g)
1-2 tablespoons apple cider vinegar, plus extra for the rice
sprinkle of dried herbs (I use herbes de Provence or a mix of dried thyme, basil, rosemary and oregano)
2 large butternut squash (2kg), cut into bite-sized cubes
olive oil
2 teaspoons paprika
1 teaspoon ground cumin
2 tablespoons nutritional yeast (see Top tip)
1 tablespoon tahini
juice of 1 lemon
handful of finely chopped fresh coriander
salt and pepper

Put the rice in a saucepan with 3½ mugs (1 litre) water and add a sprinkling of salt, a drizzle of apple cider vinegar and a sprinkle of dried herbs for some extra flavour. Bring the pan to the boil and let it bubble for 5 minutes or so, then simmer for about 45 minutes, covered, until the rice is soft, but not soggy, and all the water has evaporated. You'll need to stir the rice and may need to add more boiling water as it cooks.

Preheat the oven to 210°C (fan 190°C).

Places the squash squares onto a baking tray and drizzle with olive oil, paprika, cumin, salt and pepper. Bake for about 20–30 minutes, until the cubes are perfectly soft and delicious. Roasting the squash really brings out the flavour, making it much more delicious than if it was steamed.

Put three-quarters of the squash into a food processor with about ¼ mug (75ml) water plus the nutritional yeast, apple cider vinegar, tahini, salt and lemon juice. Blend until a smooth creamy consistency forms.

Once the rice is about 5 minutes away from being cooked, and there is very little to no water left, stir in the creamy squash mix. Then add the remaining pieces of squash and a handful of coriander to serve.

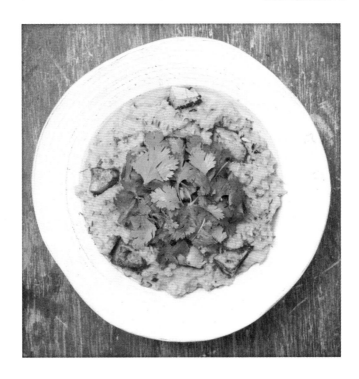

the ultimate comfort food

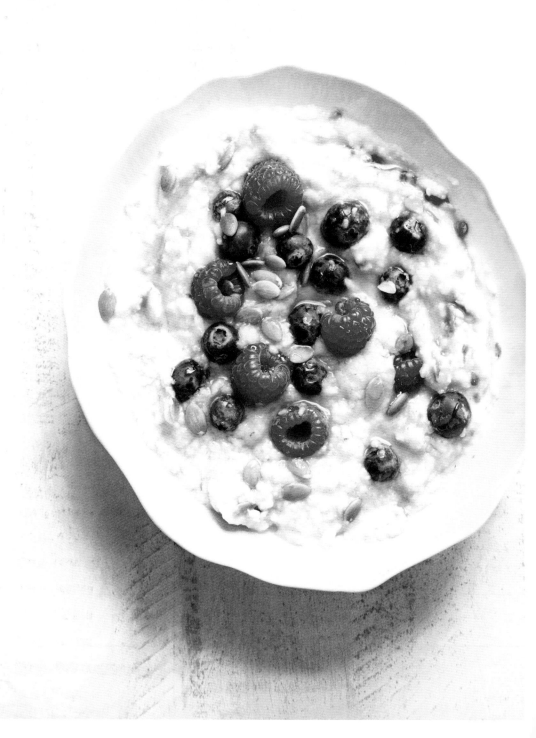

CREAMY COCONUT PORRIDGE

I might go as far as to say that this is the world's best porridge. It's just so insanely rich and creamy, yet so nourishing! It's such a speedy breakfast too and will keep you energised for hours thanks to all the goodness it has. It's been such a huge hit on the blog and I've seen hundreds and hundreds of photos of Deliciously Ella fans recreating and loving it on Instagram, so I knew this one was too good not to share in the book too. I love my bowl topped with raisins and almonds, plus some fresh blueberries and raw honey.

Serves 1

⅓ mug oats (40g)
3–4 tablespoons coconut milk
1 banana, sliced
1 tablespoon almond butter (recipe on page 24)
1 tablespoon coconut oil
big handful of almonds
big handful of raisins

Place the oats in a saucepan with ⅔ mug (200ml) water, the coconut milk and half the sliced banana.

Allow the mixture to simmer for about 10 minutes until all the liquid has been absorbed. At this point, stir in the almond butter and coconut oil and allow it to cook for another minute or two so that they totally melt into the porridge.

Meanwhile, place the almonds in a food processor and pulse for about 30 seconds until they are partially crushed. Place them in a dry frying pan for a couple of minutes to get crunchy.

Pour the cooked oats into a bowl and add the remaining slices of banana, the raisins and toasted almonds.

Top tip

If you're in a hurry in the morning, you can leave your oats to soak in the water overnight and then just cook them with the coconut milk in the morning for 2 minutes or so until it's hot, as the oats will already be soft so they won't need the normal cooking time.

APPLE AND CINNAMON PORRIDGE BAKE

I'm totally obsessed with porridge; anyone who knows me can tell you I eat it for breakfast, lunch and dinner and seem to have it almost every day! So I like to mix up my porridge combinations to keep it interesting, and baking it is one of the best ways to do that. Baking porridge really brings out the flavours of all the ingredients to create something insanely flavoursome. It tastes amazing topped with coconut yoghurt and fresh fruit at the end, or lots of raisins or goji berries and extra nut butter.

Serves 4

2 mugs oats (240g)

1½ mugs almond milk (450ml) (recipe on page 20) (oat milk and coconut milk will also work perfectly)

2 red apples

8 Medjool dates

2 teaspoons ground cinnamon

2 tablespoons honey

2 tablespoons almond butter (recipe on page 24)

Place the oats in a bowl with the almond milk and allow them to soak for 10 minutes.

While the oats soak, preheat the oven to 200°C (fan 180°C).

Peel the apples and grate them onto a plate, using the coarse side of a box grater.

Next, slice the dates in half, remove the pits, and then cut them again into eighths.

Once the oats have soaked for 10 minutes, stir in the grated apple, date chunks, cinnamon, honey and almond butter, and then pour the mix into a baking dish.

Place the dish in the oven and allow it to cook for 15–20 minutes, until all the liquid has been absorbed and the top begins to change colour.

Top tip

You can try mixing up the fruit in here too to make new variations. Adding pears or banana instead of the apples tastes amazing or you can add some berries alongside the apple for extra goodness.

APPLE AND HONEY LOAF

This Apple and Honey Loaf is quite similar to banana bread in terms of texture, but the mixture of apples and honey gives it a new exciting flavour! It's so easy to cook and makes for the best snack – it's a great thing to take to work to fight off the afternoon energy slump. I especially love it served with lots of almond butter and banana slices.

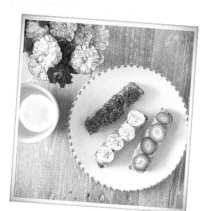

makes 1 loaf

3 heaped tablespoons apple purée
   (recipe on page 19)
6 tablespoons honey (I use raw honey)
1 ripe banana, peeled
1 mug ground almonds (120g)
1 tablespoon chia seeds
1 mug brown rice flour (200g)
coconut oil, for greasing

Preheat the oven to 200°C
(fan 180°C).

Place the apple purée, honey and banana into a large mixing bowl and mash the three together with a fork until you have a smooth mix.

Stir in the ground almonds, chia seeds, rice flour and 4 tablespoons water and mix until smooth.

Grease a standard-sized loaf tin with coconut oil before pouring the mixture in and spreading it across. It's meant to be a long loaf and only 2-3cm or so tall.

Bake for 50 minutes until the top turns a golden brown and you can pull a clean knife out of the middle of it.

Top tip

Don't try and make the loaf too thick or else it won't set; it's really only meant to be about 2–3cm thick.

BERRY SCONES WITH COCONUT CREAM

Scones and cream were always my favourite summer dessert and I really missed them for a while when I changed my diet, so I was unbelievably excited when I mastered this recipe! The scones really are so delicious and the cream is just divine; it's amazing how much you can do with such simple ingredients. I love serving these with my Strawberry Jam (page 187) and some slices of fresh strawberries.

Makes 12 scones

For the cake

2 mugs buckwheat flour (400g)
2 mugs ground almonds (240g)
1 mug almond milk (300ml)
    (recipe on page 20)
4 tablespoons maple syrup
3 tablespoons apple purée
    (recipe on page 19)
8 strawberries (250g)
½ mug blueberries (100g)
coconut oil, for greasing

For the coconut cream

200g coconut cream (coconut
    cream comes in sachets and is
    totally solid – coconut milk is
    not a substitute here)
strawberry jam, to serve (recipe
    on page 187)

For the cake

Preheat the oven to 180°C (fan 160°C).

Place the buckwheat flour, ground almonds, almond milk, maple syrup and apple purée in a large mixing bowl and stir until smooth.

Slice the strawberries into tiny pieces and stir them, and the blueberries, into the mix.

Grease two baking trays with the coconut oil and then scoop the mixture out and form into round scone shapes on the trays.

Bake for 35–40 minutes until the tops turn a golden brown.

Remove the scones from the oven and allow them to cool.

For the coconut cream

Place the bag of coconut cream in a mug of boiling water and allow it to melt.

Once the cream has melted, place it into a large mixing bowl with 3 tablespoons water and whisk it until it's nice and creamy.

To serve, cut the scones open and top with coconut cream and strawberry jam.

Top tip

Don't try and freeze the coconut cream, I've tried this a few times and every time you warm it up, it ends up lumpy and very unappetising – it's a great excuse to finish any leftovers off!

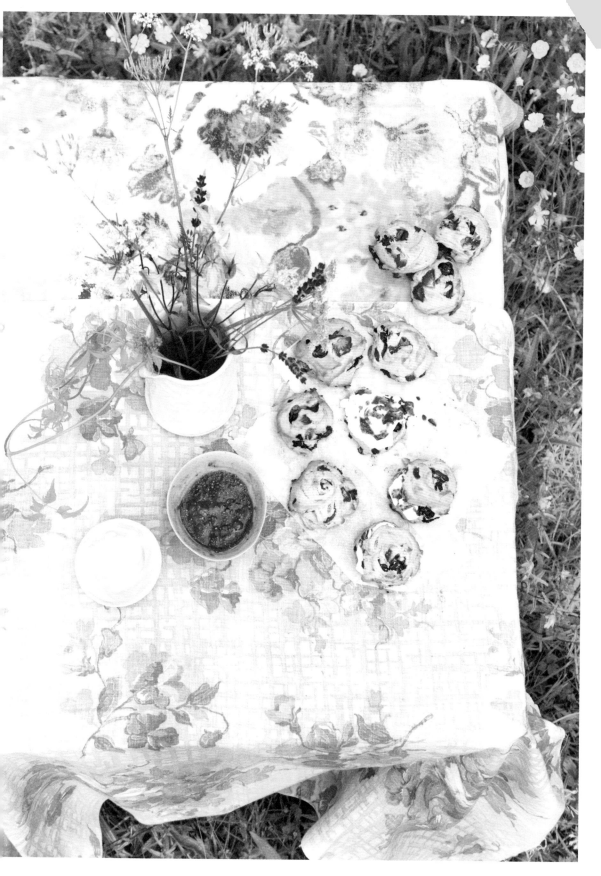

SIMPLE OAT COOKIES

These cookies couldn't be any simpler to make, which is awesome. They're all about celebrating simple, healthy goodness using all your store cupboard ingredients, plus some ripe bananas. They're a delicious thing to keep in your kitchen during the week for those times when you need something sweet. If you're after something extra specially good, try pairing these with my Cacao and Hazelnut Spread (page 79) – it's absolute heaven!

makes 10 large cookies

3 large, ripe bananas (400g)
4 heaped tablespoons almond butter (recipe on page 24)
1 tablespoon coconut oil, plus extra for greasing
4 tablespoons maple syrup
1½ mugs oats (180g)

Preheat the oven to 200°C (fan 180°).

Peel the bananas and place them in a large mixing bowl. Mash them with a fork until they're smooth.

Add the almond butter, coconut oil and maple syrup to the mashed bananas and mix well until a sticky mix forms, at which point, stir in the oats.

Once the oats are totally covered and nicely sticky, grease a baking tray with coconut oil and then scoop heaped tablespoons of the mixture onto the tray, using your hands to spread them out into cookie shapes. They should be quite nice and thin so that they become crunchy.

Once all the cookies are on the tray, place it into the oven and bake for 18–20 minutes, until the cookies begin to turn a golden brown.

Remove the cookies from the oven and allow them to cool for about 5 minutes before enjoying.

Store these in an airtight container at room temperature.

FLAPJACKS

These are quite similar to the Simple Oat Cookies (page 62) in that they're very s[...]
make and use your store cupboard essentials. They're also totally delicious and a g[...]
to keep in your kitchen. I love this kind of dessert too as it's sweet, but not at all sickly. These
make a great afternoon or mid-morning snack as they're full of fibre and plant protein so
you'll feel satisfied and energised for hours and hours!

makes about 20 flapjacks

3 mugs oats (360g)
2 bananas (200g)
6 tablespoons maple syrup
6 tablespoons cashew butter (or any nut butter works)
4 tablespoons coconut oil, plus extra for greasing

Preheat the oven to 200°C (fan 180°C).

Place the oats into a mixing bowl.

Mash the bananas with a fork and add them to a saucepan with the maple
syrup, cashew butter and coconut oil. Allow it to simmer until it forms a
liquid.

Pour the liquid over the oats and stir well so that they're fully covered.

Grease a baking tray with the coconut oil. Transfer the flapjack mix into the
baking tray, pressing it down firmly with a spatula so that it's very compact.

Bake for 15–20 minutes until the top starts to
brown.

Once it's cooked, take the tray out of the oven and
leave it to fully cool before slicing the flapjacks up.

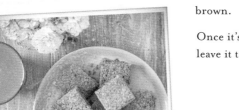

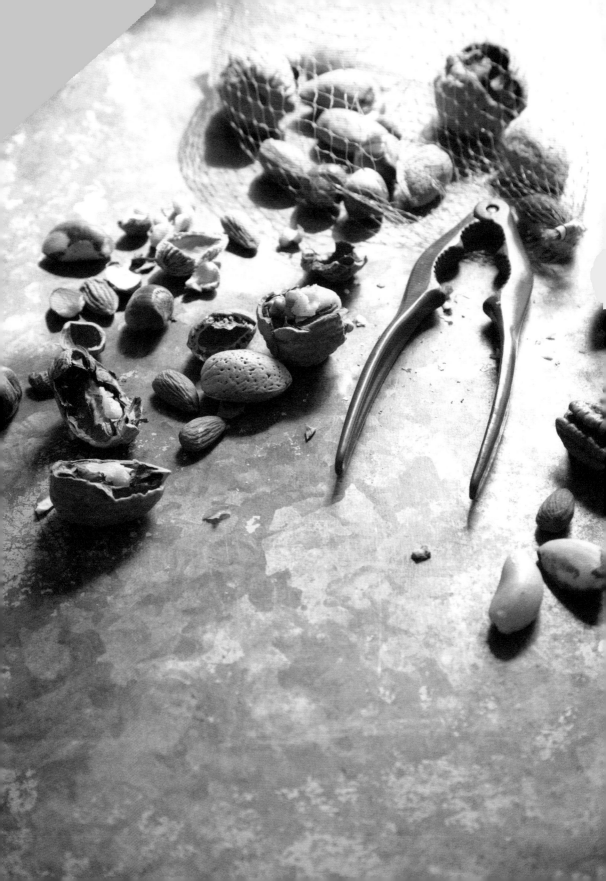

NUTS AND SEEDS
small and amazingly versatile

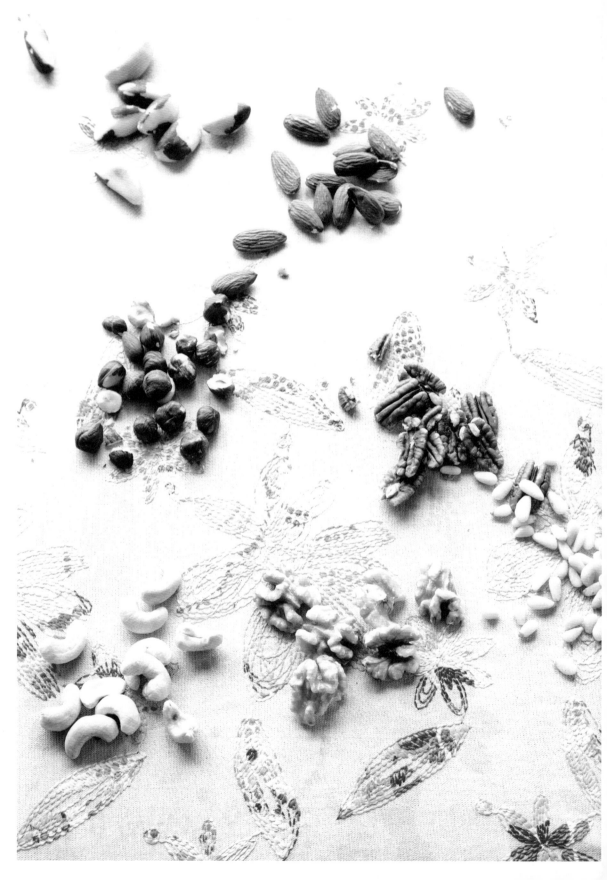

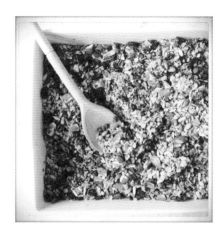

nuts and seeds

I'm obsessed with both nuts and seeds. They're absolutely incredible as they taste amazing and they're packed with so much goodness that nourishes every part of our bodies. I try to add them to every meal in some way, shape or form. The great thing about them is that whilst they taste amazing on their own and make delicious snacks, they can also be used to make a million other things, some of which you wouldn't normally think of. They work so well in obvious things like Granola (page 76) and Granola Bars (page 75) or for toppings for yoghurts and salads and as ingredients in cookies or crackers, but they can also be used in more inventive ways to make awesome dishes from Superfood Bread (page 80) to Raw Brownies (page 89) and Double-Layered Hazelnut Cake (page 92). Nuts can also be used to make nut milk, which is so simple to prepare (page 20), and all nuts and seeds can be ground down into flours, which can then be used as the basis for almost anything – it's an easy way to make things gluten-free and really healthy.

I know that lots of people are nervous of nuts because of their fat content, so they stay away from them, but they're actually an amazing part of a healthy diet and we really shouldn't look at the calories. Besides, all calories really aren't created equal – a handful of nuts just isn't the same as a Mars Bar, and that's a very important thing to hold on to when you start to eat a very natural diet. Of course each different variety of nut has its own awesome benefits, but they're all filled with incredible plant protein, healthy fats, vitamins and minerals, all of which we need to look and feel our best. Honestly, I was pretty nervous of them when I started eating this way too, but after a while I realised that they were really helping to heal my energy issues and my skin was getting cleaner, my hair shinier and my nails stronger, which together quickly dispelled all fears and I became a nut-addict! I now get through a jar of nut butter every couple of days, it's my absolute favourite snack, and I'm so much healthier for it.

I know that nut allergies can be an issue though, so I want to talk a little bit about that. I've tried to make lots of nut-free recipes for you throughout the book so hopefully there are still lots of delicious things for you to make. If you have an allergy to one kind of nut though, you can always switch it with another one (bear in mind as you go through the book that all the nuts in every recipe are completely interchangeable – of course this may cause subtle differences in the taste and texture of the dish but nothing major at all), so please feel free to swap in the nut that works best for you.

Alternatively, you can swap the nut for pumpkin seeds. This changes the taste and texture a little more, but it still works in recipes where the nut is just one of a few ingredients, such as in the Brazil Nut and Rocket Pesto (page 86) for example, the Raw Brownies (page 89) or Almond and Chia Energy Bites (page 72). It is tricky, though, to switch seeds into recipes that contain a few different types of nuts, like the Superfood Bread (page 80) or recipes where the nuts are needed to make something creamy, like the Creamy Brazil Nut Cheese (page 85) or Cacao and Hazelnut Spread (page 79).

Each nut does have its own awesome characteristics though, and once you know all about these, it should help to explain why I use certain nuts in certain recipes. This should also help you work out the best substitutions if you need them.

I store my nuts in glass airtight containers so

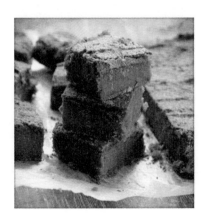

that they stay fresh for ages. It's really important to keep them in something airtight otherwise they can go rancid. They can live at room temperature though, so you don't need to worry about them taking up too much space in your fridge. When buying them, always go for the unsalted, unroasted nuts. You want totally plain nuts that are one hundred per cent nut, with no added oils or preservatives. This is really important for all the recipes throughout the book.

If you're snacking on nuts, you can absolutely roast them. Just place them in a 180°C (fan 160°C) oven with some salt and a drizzling of olive oil and roast for about 15 minutes, or until they have a great crunch.

ALMONDS

Almonds are without any doubt the nut that I use the most. I find they're the most versatile, and their flavour goes with just about everything. They're a real beauty food too as they're packed with vitamin E, which is the most important vitamin for glowing skin, so they're really an amazing addition to your life. Plus, there's lots of calcium in almonds, which is essential for strong bones and teeth. I use ground almonds in most of my baking, especially in cakes and my Superfood Bread (page 80). They're amazing crushed in a food processor too and then used in raw desserts, as in my Key Lime Pie (page 196) and Berry Cheesecake (page 193).

I also love almond milk and make a batch every week to use in my smoothies, granola, porridge and baking. I've included my almond milk recipe in the Getting Started chapter (page 20). Almonds aren't as creamy as cashews or brazil nuts, so they're not great in things like nut cheese, cheesecakes or pesto as you won't get quite the same consistency. I find the best substitution for almonds are pecans as the texture is quite similar; you'll just get a more caramel-like flavour, which is pretty delicious.

BRAZIL NUTS

Brazil nuts are much chunkier than almonds, which means they add a whole lot of creaminess to anything, as you'll find in the Brazil Nut and Rocket Pesto Pasta (page 86) or the Creamy Brazil Nut Cheese (page 85). In this way, they're pretty similar to cashews, but they're much more savoury in flavour so they work better in main dishes rather than desserts, which is why they're my nut of choice in things like pesto or nut cheese. That being said, if you have a brazil nut allergy, then using cashews is still perfect as a substitution. Like almonds and most other nuts, they're a great source of vitamin E, as well as monounsaturated fats, but the thing that's special about brazil nuts is their selenium. Selenium is a mineral that we're often short of, but it's essential for immune and thyroid function and brazil nuts are full of it.

CASHEWS

So cashews are the brazil nuts of desserts: sweet, creamy and totally delicious. If you soak them for a few hours in a bowl of water and then blend them, you'll get something really divine (you want to drain the water first though). They're an amazing addition to smoothies too for the same reason, making them taste a bit like a milkshake! That's not to say that you can't use them in savoury dishes; you absolutely can. I love them chopped and toasted before being sprinkled onto salads, like in my side dish of Broccoli with a Tahini Dressing (page 159) and stir-fries, where they add a sweet, crunchy touch. In terms of substitutions, cashews are always best replaced with brazil nuts.

HAZELNUTS

For me, hazelnuts really only have one association – Nutella! I know that's very unoriginal of me, but when I taste or smell hazelnuts, it's really the first and last thing I think about! Of course, I've included my healthy Cacao and Hazelnut Spread here for you (page 79), which tastes

just as delicious. It tastes amazing spread over my Superfood Bread (page 80), mixed into my Creamy Coconut Porridge (page 57) or used as a dip for fruit. There's just such a strong link between hazelnuts and chocolate, and to be honest I haven't come up with many savoury hazelnut recipes yet, as I get so obsessed with the sweet ones – Double-Layered Hazelnut Cake being the best (page 92)! Their texture isn't dissimilar to that of almonds, so if you can't eat hazelnuts, then you can replace them with almonds.

PECANS

I find that pecans taste a little bit like caramel. When they're roasted, the flavour comes out even more and it really feels like you're eating candy – especially if you've added a little maple syrup and cinnamon to the mix, as in my favourite Cinnamon and Pecan Granola (page 76). Like almonds, they work really well when they're ground down into a flour, so they're amazing for baking. As with all the other nuts, you can also make nut milk from pecans, although it's not my favourite as they're not that fleshy, so you need so many of them to make milk, plus their skin doesn't make it as smooth as milk from blanched almonds, brazil nuts or cashews. Pecans are full of heart-healthy monounsaturated fats, including oleic acid, which help to lower cholesterol and prevent heart and cardiovascular disease.

PINE NUTS

Pine nuts are actually a seed, not a nut, and I use them in a similar way to pumpkin or sunflower seeds. They're more of a topping to add extra flavour to recipes, like my Warm Winter Salad (page 154). They're my favourite of all the seeds though, as they have such a delicious texture, especially after they've been toasted, which makes them half crunchy and half soft. They're also deliciously sweet with a pretty strong flavour that really adds to whatever you pair it with. I love sprinkling them over soups and salads and, of course, using them to make pesto. If you can't eat pine nuts, pumpkin seeds make an amazing replacement. Like almonds, pine nuts are a great source of vitamin E, so they're good for your skin, plus they have lots of B vitamins, which are so important for energy.

PUMPKIN SEEDS

Pumpkin seeds are pretty awesomely versatile too. I don't think they taste quite as nice on their own as pine nuts do as they're a little sharper, but they're great mixed into anything as they have such a great crunch and their flavour isn't strong enough for you to notice it. They're an important ingredient in healthy baking, from Superfood Bread (page 80) to Granola (page 76) and they also make the best nut replacement in baking. They're delicious toasted with a little chilli and paprika or just sprinkled raw onto salads, risottos, quinoa dishes, porridge and smoothie bowls. Plus pumpkin seeds are a fantastic source of goodness, especially antioxidants, which are great for glowing skin; zinc, which is so important for metabolising and processing carbohydrates, fat and protein; and manganese, which is important for just about everything, including strengthening your bones and regulating your blood sugar.

SUNFLOWER SEEDS

Sunflower seeds aren't the most exciting, but they're really good for us as they're full of vitamins, minerals and protein. I love them as they add a great crunch to whatever you're eating. So, like pumpkin seeds, they're great to sprinkle over just about anything. They also have a lovely texture – it's firm, but still tender – so they go with just about anything and are great in savoury baking for things like crackers and bread. Sunflower seeds are a serious beauty food too as they're packed with vitamin E, which is essential for beautiful skin.

CHIA SEEDS

Chia seeds belong in their own category really, as whilst they are technically a seed, you use them in a very different way to pumpkin or sunflower seeds. In terms of what they look and taste like, there's not much to say as they are basically just little black dots, which don't really have any natural flavour, but in terms of what they can do, they are actually little pieces of magic.

Chia seeds are an amazing ingredient in cooking as when mixed with any liquid, they expand to about ten times their original size, making a gluey mix that binds into a gel so it holds whatever you're cooking together really well. They're good as egg-replacement binders in baking, as you'll find in recipes like the Apple and Honey Loaf (page 59) and for thickening things up, as in the Chia Breakfast Pudding (page 74).

The other reason to use them is that they're insanely good for us and as they're so small, you can add them to virtually anything without noticing that they're there. They're absolutely bursting with fibre, which keeps you energised and satisfied for hours, as well as omega-3 fatty acids, which are very anti-inflammatory and are amazing for glowing skin. They're also a great source of calcium, which we all know is crucial for strong bones, as well as protein and iron, which are both vital for energy. If you're nervous of using them, start by simply adding a couple of teaspoons to your morning smoothie and you'll soon find that they'll make you feel amazing and you won't even realise that they're there.

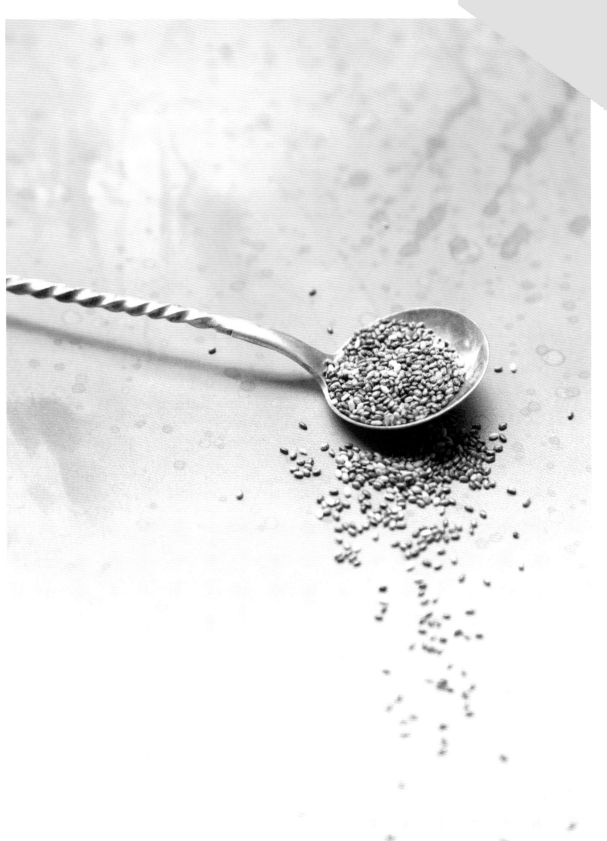

energy bites are based on one of the most popular recipes from my blog. I've been making them almost every week for the last few years and they've done wonders to keep my energy going, even when I'm at my busiest! They're wonderfully sweet thanks to the dates, while the cacao makes them amazingly chocolaty and then the almonds, almond butter, coconut oil and chia seeds give you all the goodness you need to stay energised. They last for ages too, so you can make big batches and store them in the fridge so that you always have a sweet snack on hand. Plus, they travel well, so you can take them to work with you too.

makes about 20 balls

1 mug almonds (200g)

2 mugs Medjool dates (400g)

4 tablespoons raw cacao powder

2 tablespoons almond butter (recipe on page 24)

2 tablespoons coconut oil

2 tablespoons chia seeds

Start by putting the almonds in a food processor and whiz for about 30 seconds, until they're nicely crushed.

Then pit the dates and add them, plus all the other ingredients and 2 tablespoons water, to the processor and blend again until everything has mixed together perfectly and it's all nice and sticky.

Roll the mix into balls.

Place the balls in the freezer for an hour to set, then store in an airtight container in the fridge.

Top tip

If you don't have any almonds, try swapping them for any other nuts. You can also add things like hemp protein or maca if you want to give more goodness to each bite.

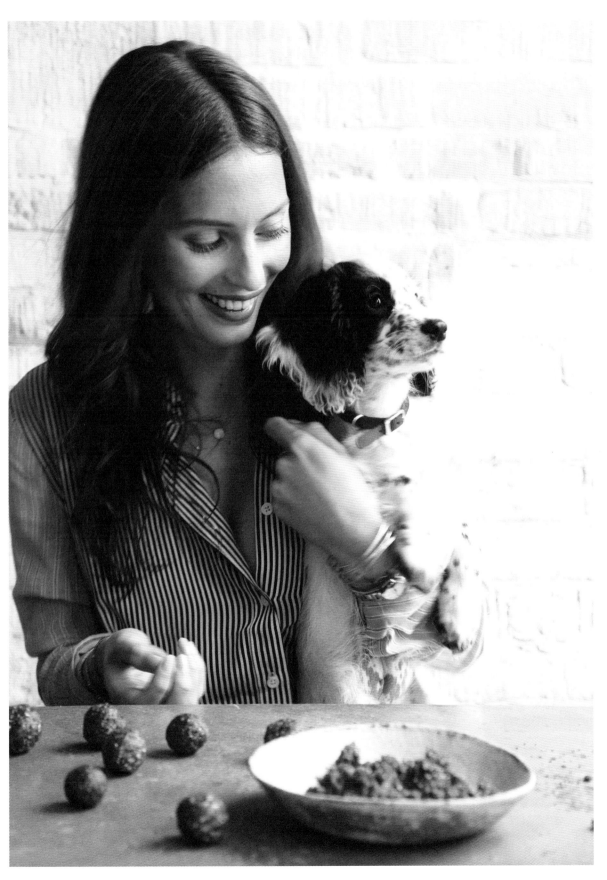

CHIA BREAKFAST PUDDING

This Chia Breakfast Pudding is incredible if you're busy and don't have time to make breakfast as it's made the night before, so you can just grab it and go in the morning. The chia seeds expand overnight to absorb all the flavours of the pudding, so each bite bursts with sweet scents of banana, blueberries and honey, while the almond butter and almond milk make it wonderfully creamy.

Serves 1

1 mug almond milk (300ml) (recipe on page 20)
1 ripe banana, peeled
1 tablespoon almond butter (recipe on page 24)
1 teaspoon honey or maple syrup
handful of frozen blueberries
5 tablespoons chia seeds

Place the almond milk, banana, almond butter, honey and frozen blueberries in a blender and blend until smooth and creamy.

Pour the mix into a glass and stir in the chia seeds.

Cover the glass and leave it in the fridge overnight, or for at least 6 hours, so that it sets and the chia seeds expand.

Either enjoy the breakfast pudding as it is or top the glass off with fresh fruit and granola.

Top tip
Keep this interesting by changing the blueberries for a different fruit every now and again. I love using either mango, strawberries or pineapple.

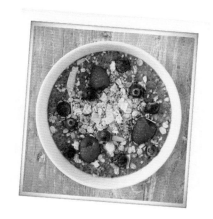

GRANOLA BARS

When you start eating healthily it's really important to keep delicious, healthy snacks in your kitchen so that you always have something nutritious on hand to enjoy, which should stop you from reaching towards the processed snacks. These Granola Bars are a great option for this as they're easy to make, they taste amazing and they're full of protein and fibre, which will give you lots of energy and keep you feeling satisfied for hours so you won't be craving processed sugar!

Makes about 20 bars
20 Medjool dates (350g)
I mug sunflower seeds (175g)
I mug pumpkin seeds (175g)
I mug flaxseeds (200g)
I mug raisins (200g)
2 mugs oats (240g)
3 tablespoons chia seeds
3 tablespoons ground cinnamon

Preheat the oven to 180°C (fan 160°C).

Pit the dates, then place them in a saucepan with 2 mugs (600ml) boiling water and simmer for 5 minutes, until they are really soft.

While the dates cook, place the sunflower seeds, pumpkin seeds, flaxseeds, raisins and oats in a large mixing bowl.

Once the dates have cooked for 5 minutes, place them and the remaining water from the pan in a blender with the chia seeds and cinnamon. Blend until smooth.

Pour the date purée over the oats and seed mix and stir thoroughly until everything is coated and sticky.

Grease a large 40 x 28cm baking tray with coconut oil, then pour in the granola and press it down firmly so that it is tightly packed and smooth on the top.

Bake for 30–40 minutes, until the top starts to turn a golden brown. After 20 minutes though, remove from the oven and cut into bars, then place them back in to finish cooking.

Top tip
Try taking a couple of these in your bag so that you can enjoy them whenever you're feeling tired.

CINNAMON PECAN GRANOLA

This granola is one of my oldest and most loved recipes. I just love the nutty, crunchy texture and the sweet echoes of maple, cinnamon and coconut. Eating a big bowl of this for breakfast with home-made almond milk (page 20) and some fresh berries makes me feel so awesome! It's delicious sprinkled over baked fruit too – like a speedy crumble!

Makes 1 large container of granola

1 mug pecans (180g)
½ mug almonds (100g)
2 mugs oats (240g)
1 mug pumpkin seeds (175g)
1 mug sunflower seeds (175g)
½ mug flaxseeds (100g)
3 tablespoons coconut oil
3 tablespoons maple syrup
3 teaspoons ground cinnamon
1 mug raisins (200g)

Preheat the oven to 200°C (fan 180°C).

Place the pecans and almonds in a food processor and pulse for about 30 seconds so that they are partially crushed. Then add them to a large mixing bowl with all the other dry ingredients, except the raisins and cinnamon, and stir together.

Next, melt the coconut oil with the maple syrup and cinnamon on the stove. Once it has dissolved into a sweet liquid, add it to the dry bowl and mix well. This should form a delicious oaty, nutty bowl, which is slightly sticky.

Place the mixture into a baking tray and bake for 30–40 minutes until crunchy. During this time you'll need to stir the mixture to ensure that every bit of the granola gets nicely toasted and the top doesn't burn.

Once the granola is cooked perfectly, remove the tray from the oven and allow it to cool, then stir in the raisins. Store the granola in an airtight container.

Top tip

If you don't have any pecans then you can use any other nuts. You can also replace the raisins with dried apricots, goji berries or pieces of dates.

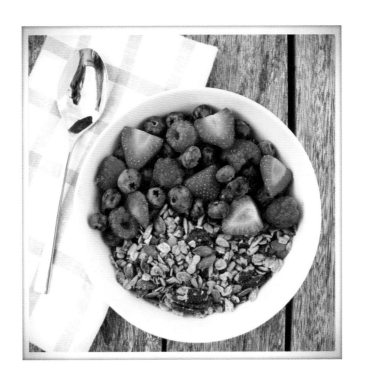

the perfect breakfast?

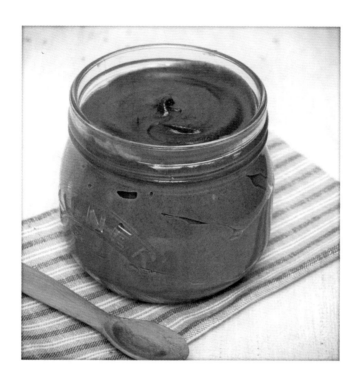

one of my favourite things!

CACAO AND HAZELNUT SPREAD

You'll feel so much better eating this spread, both your taste buds and your tummy will be singing with happiness! It is really full of goodness and it tastes incredible too. I love spreading this over my Simple Oat Cookies (page 62) or enjoying it with my Berry Scones with Coconut Cream (page 60). It also works really well as a sweet dip for fruit – try dunking apple slices into your jar for a great snack or easy dessert.

Makes 1 big jar
2 mugs hazelnuts (375g)
½ mug maple syrup (150ml)
3 tablespoons raw cacao powder

Preheat the oven to 200°C (fan 180°C).

Bake the hazelnuts for about 10 minutes, then take them out of the oven and allow them to cool.

Once cool, place them in a food processor and blend for about 10 minutes, until they totally break down. Then add the maple syrup and cacao and blend again, before gradually pouring in ½ mug (150ml) water (it's important that the first three are properly mixed before you add the water though).

Top tip
You really need a strong processor for this recipe, otherwise it just won't come out that smoothly.

SUPERFOOD BREAD

This Superfood Bread is a staple in my life. I always have a few slices of it in my freezer as it's the basis of my favourite five-minute meal. I love toasting it and then topping it with lots of creamy avocado, home-made Hummus (page 102), roasted tomato slices and a sprinkling of seeds or bean sprouts for a crunch. It's also amazing dunked into soup or eaten with a salad to make the meal a little heartier. You can make a few loaves at once, slice them up and then freeze the slices so that you can just pull a few pieces out when you need them.

makes 1 loaf

1 mug almonds (200g)
1½ mugs pumpkin seeds (260g)
1 mug brown rice flour (200g)
½ mug sunflower seeds (85g)
3 tablespoons psyllium husk powder (see Top tip)
3 tablespoons dried mixed herbs (I like herbes de Provence)
2 tablespoons chia seeds
salt and pepper

Place the almonds and 1 mug of the pumpkin seeds in a food processor and blend until a flour forms.

Pour the flour in a large mixing bowl with all the dry ingredients and mix well.

Add in 2 mugs (600ml) cold water, stirring the whole mixture together.

Leave the bowl to one side for about an hour, at which point all the water should have been absorbed and the mix will be totally stuck together.

After an hour, preheat the oven to 200°C (fan 180°C). Turn the dough out onto a baking tray. Don't try and make this loaf too thick or else it won't set properly, it's only meant to be 5–7cm tall.

Bake the bread for about 45 minutes, until the top turns a golden brown and you can pull a clean knife out of the middle.

Top tip

With the psyllium husk powder, there is no substitution as this holds the loaf together. You can find it online or in health-food stores.

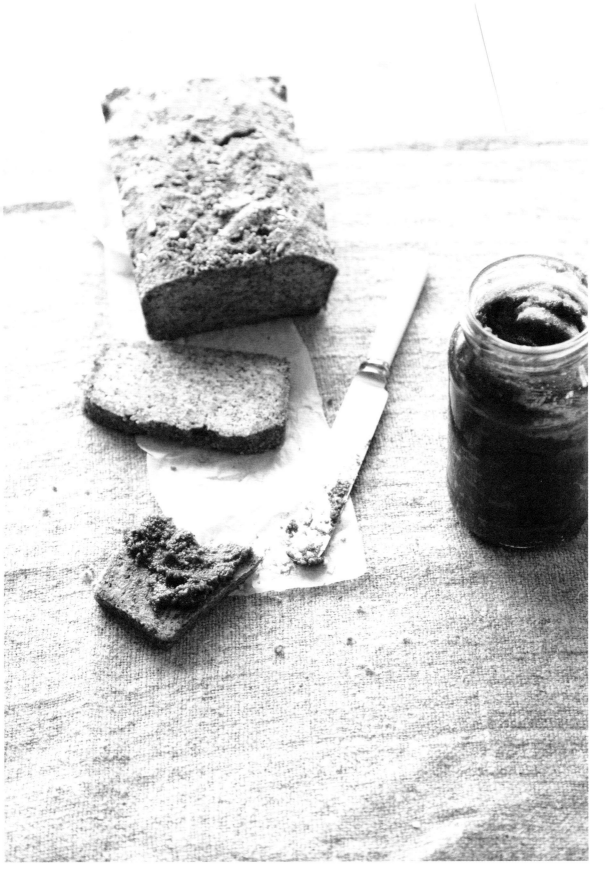

SUPERFOOD CRACKERS

These crackers are the best way to use your juice pulp so that you don't waste any of your veggies! They're so easy to make too and they're so versatile. I love dunking them into pots of my Creamy Brazil Nut Cheese (page 85) or my home-made Guacamole (page 159), or breaking them into pieces and sprinkling them over salads and soups for a little extra crunch. You can spice these up a little too by adding extra ingredients. I like chopping up sun-dried tomatoes and olives with fresh rosemary and sprinkling them into the mix.

makes about 20 crackers

200g juice pulp (I like carrot, apple and ginger pulp)
1 mug ground almonds (120g)
½ mug sunflower seeds (85g)
½ mug pumpkin seeds (85g)
3 tablespoons olive oil
1 tablespoon tahini
1 tablespoon tamari
salt and pepper

Preheat the oven to 110°C (fan 90°C).

Simply place all the ingredients into a mixing bowl and stir them together until the mix is sticky.

Pour the mixture onto a flat baking tray lined with baking paper, then use a spatula to press it down so that it's nice and thin and very compact.

Bake for an hour and a half, until crispy.

Store at room temperature in an airtight container.

Top tip

If you don't have any pulp from a juicer, then you can grate 200g worth of carrots instead.

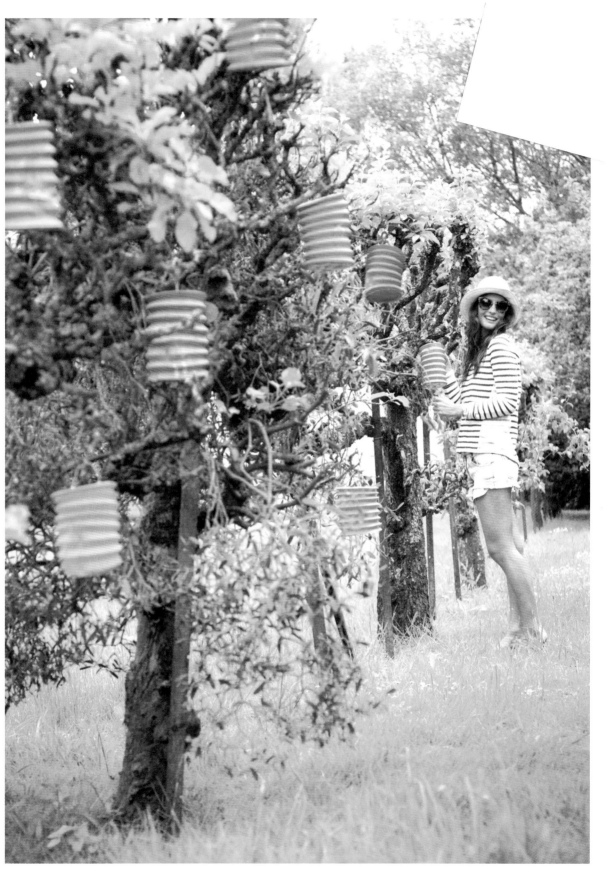

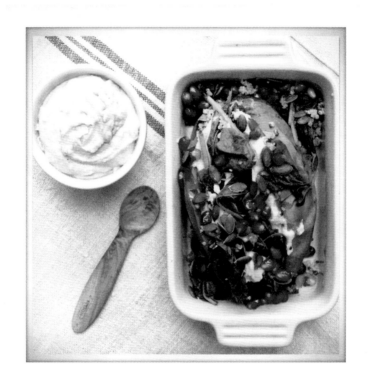

sounds strange – tastes delicious!

CREAMY BRAZIL NUT CHEESE

This is a great side dish that adds taste and texture to any meal as it's so creamy with a wonderful nutty taste. I love adding it to a pile of stir-fried veggies (page 143) or spreading it over a baked sweet potato with a side of Marinated Kale Salad (page 153). It also works really well as a dip for crudités and can be added to salad for a creamy protein boost.

makes 1 bowl

1 lemon
couple of fresh rosemary sprigs
2 teaspoons nutritional yeast (see Top tip)
1 mug brazil nuts (120g)
1 tablespoon olive oil
salt and pepper

Simply juice the lemon and pull the rosemary leaves off the sprigs, then add them to a food processor with the nutritional yeast, brazil nuts, olive oil, salt and pepper and whiz until combined.

Store any leftovers in an airtight container in the fridge.

Top tip

Nutritional yeast is not the same as baker's yeast that's used in bread, so watch out for that! Nutritional yeast is available in health-food stores and online. It's a deactivated strain of yeast that tastes like cheese, which is why I use it in this recipe, but if you don't have any, then don't worry, it still tastes delicious without it.

BRAZIL NUT AND ROCKET PESTO PASTA

This pasta is my favourite dish to serve to girlfriends when they come over for an easy kitchen supper. It's simple to make, totally delicious and wonderfully comforting. It's also full of amazing green veggies, so it will give you lots of goodness. The home-made pesto here is incredible, the brazil nuts and avocado really make it so creamy, while the rocket and lemon add a slightly sharp edge that makes each bite sing with flavour.

Serves 4

1 mug brazil nuts (120g)
½ mug pine nuts (50g)
1½ avocados
2 big handfuls of rocket (50g)
big handful of fresh basil leaves (30g)
juice of 1½ lemons
8 tablespoons olive oil, plus extra for the veggies
500g penne pasta
2 courgettes
1 head of broccoli
1½ mugs peas (225g)
salt and pepper

Place the brazil nuts and pine nuts in a food processor and whiz for about a minute until they're completely crushed. At this point, add the avocado flesh, rocket, basil leaves, lemon juice, olive oil, 8 tablespoons water and the salt and pepper. Blend again until you have a smooth, creamy pesto.

Next, cook the pasta.

While the pasta cooks, chop the courgettes into thin slices and the broccoli into bite-sized pieces and place together in a frying pan with a little olive oil, salt and pepper. Sauté for 5–7 minutes until they're perfectly cooked.

While these cook, place the peas into a saucepan of cold water and cook them until the water boils, then drain them.

Finally, once the pasta has finished cooking and has been drained, toss the pasta together with the pesto, peas and sautéed veggies.

Top tip

Try making double the quantity of pesto and keep the other half in the fridge to stir into your next meal. It's great to liven up your grains and veggies or to use with crudités when you need a snack.

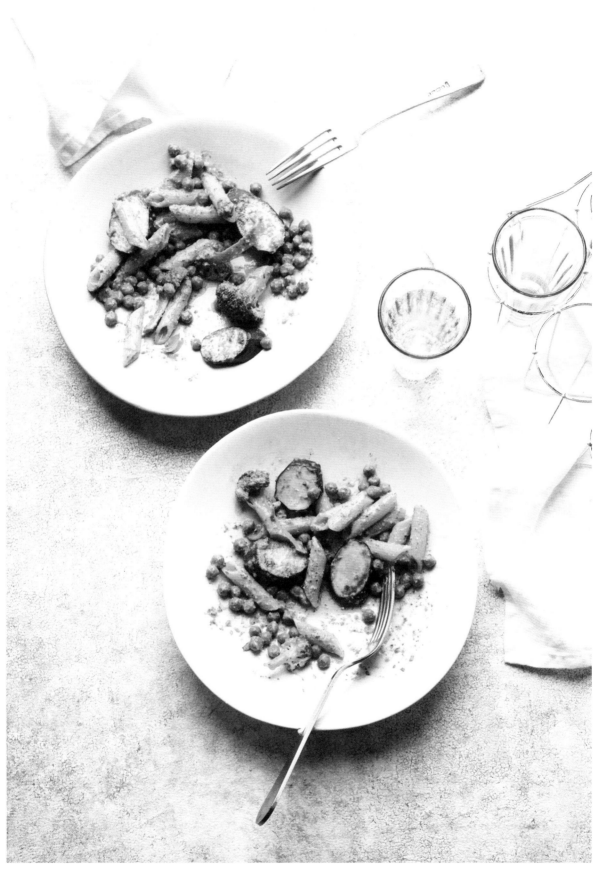

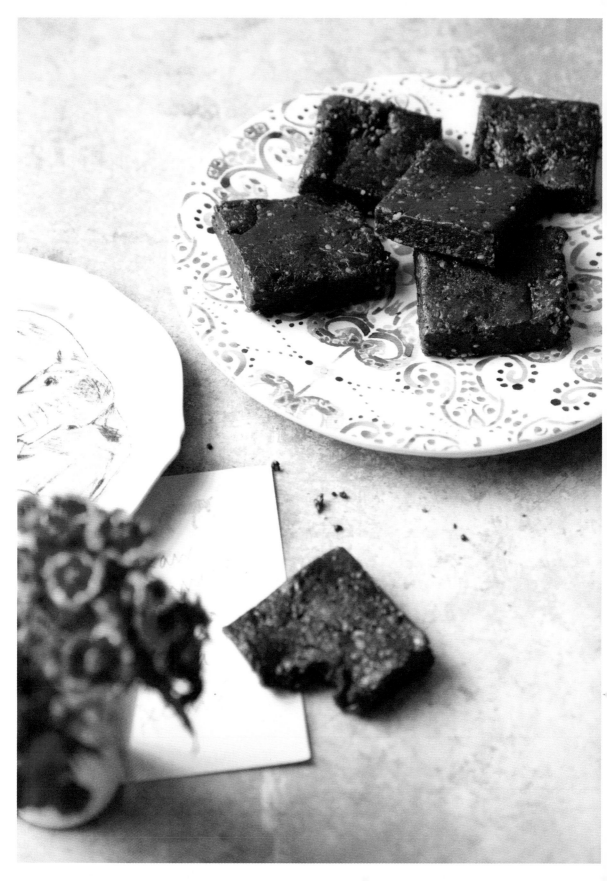

RAW BROWNIES

These brownies were my first ever blog post and my first successful attempt at creating sweet, delicious, healthy desserts – so I absolutely had to include them in the book! I'm still obsessed with them 3 years on too, as they're just so gooey and rich, and I have to admit that I normally eat at least half of the mix straight out of the food processor! They're simpler and quicker to make than the sweet potato brownies, as they require only three ingredients, which is great.

Makes 10–15 brownies

1 mug pecans (140g)
2 mugs Medjool dates (400g), pitted
3 tablespoons raw cacao powder
Optional: 2 tablespoons maple syrup

Simply pulse the pecans in a food processor until they form a crumbly mixture, then add the dates, cacao and maple syrup, if using, and blend again.

Once the mixture is very sticky, take it out of the processor and put it into a baking tray.

Freeze the brownies for an hour to let them set and then store them in the fridge.

Top tip

If you don't have any pecans, then almonds work really well too, and if you're allergic to nuts, then use sunflower seeds instead. The sweetener is totally optional in this recipe and if you'd rather use honey or agave instead of maple syrup, then that's great too.

CHOCOLATE CHIA COOKIES

This recipe is another favourite from the blog; it has consistently been one of the most popular recipes on there, so I thought you'd all love to see it in here too! These cookies are so perfectly crunchy, which I love as it makes them so satisfying. They taste amazing on their own, but they're even more incredible with my Banana Ice Cream (page 198) or dunked into my Cacao and Hazelnut Spread (page 79).

Makes 12–15 cookies

1 mug almonds (200g)

1 mug hazelnuts (190g)

1 mug buckwheat or quinoa flour (200g)

⅓ mug maple syrup (100ml)

5 Medjool dates, pitted

3 heaped tablespoons raw cacao powder

3 tablespoons chia seeds

2 tablespoons coconut oil

Preheat the oven to 200°C (fan 180°C).

Simply place the nuts into a food processor and blend for a minute or two until a flour forms, then add all of the remaining ingredients with ¼ mug (75ml) water and blend again until a sticky cookie dough forms.

Scoop about a tablespoon of the mixture into your hands, roll it into a ball and then flatten it using a spatula onto a baking tray so it is nice and thin. Keep doing this until all the cookies are on the tray.

Bake for about 20 minutes until the cookies are firm and starting to slightly brown. Then leave them to cool for a few minutes before enjoying.

Top tip

If you don't have any raw cacao powder, then you can use cocoa powder instead; you'll just need to double the quantity used as it's not as strong in flavour.

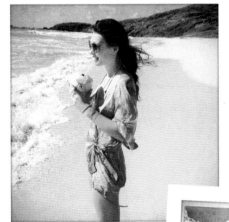

'Thank you for your amazing recipes. Deliciously Ella has changed my life. I am now a balanced, healthy happy woman who enjoys eating rather than does so full of guilt and worry.' - Nicola

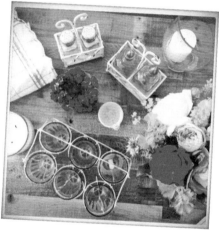

DOUBLE-LAYERED HAZELNUT CAKE

This might be the most decadent recipe in my book; it's actually pretty insane. It's made up of two layers of hazelnut and cacao-infused sponge drowned in a sea of hazelnut and coconut icing, which acts like a mix between custard and icing and really makes the cake one of the most delicious things I've ever eaten! It's one of the more expensive recipes to put together, so I save it for special celebrations and birthdays, as it really is beyond delicious. I love serving it with a side of Banana Ice Cream (page 198) and some berries.

Serves 12

For the cake

3 large ripe bananas (340g)
1½ mugs almond milk (450ml)
   (recipe on page 20)
6 tablespoons raw cacao powder
⅔ mug maple syrup (200ml)
6 tablespoons coconut palm sugar
3 mugs brown rice or buckwheat
   flour (600g)
1 mug hazelnuts (190g)
coconut oil, for greasing

For the icing

2 ripe bananas
6 tablespoons coconut palm sugar
6 tablespoons hazelnut butter
   (recipe on page 24)
2 tablespoons coconut oil

Top tip

Make the icing on its own and use it as a dip for fruit if you're after something sweet without needing any preparation time.

For the cake

Preheat the oven to 200°C (fan 180°C).

Place the ripe bananas, almond milk, raw cacao, maple syrup and coconut palm sugar in a blender and blend until smooth.

Pour the mix into a large mixing bowl and then stir in the rice flour.

Add the hazelnuts to a food processor and whiz for 30 seconds or so until they're totally crushed, but not completely smooth – like a chunky flour. Stir the crushed hazelnuts into the mixing bowl with everything else.

Grease two 20–25cm cake tins with the coconut oil before evenly distributing the mix between the two.

Place the cakes in the oven and bake for 30 minutes, until the cakes are totally cooked and you can stick a knife into the middle of them and bring it out clean.

Remove the cakes from the oven and allow them to cool for 10–15 minutes before icing them.

For the icing

While the cakes cook, place all of the icing ingredients into a blender with ½ mug (150ml) water and blend until smooth, then pour the mix into a bowl and leave it to thicken in the fridge while the cakes cool.

Once the cakes are cool, ice them separately all over, then leave them to stand for 5–10 minutes for the icing to set a little. Place one cake on top of the other and pour any extra icing on top.

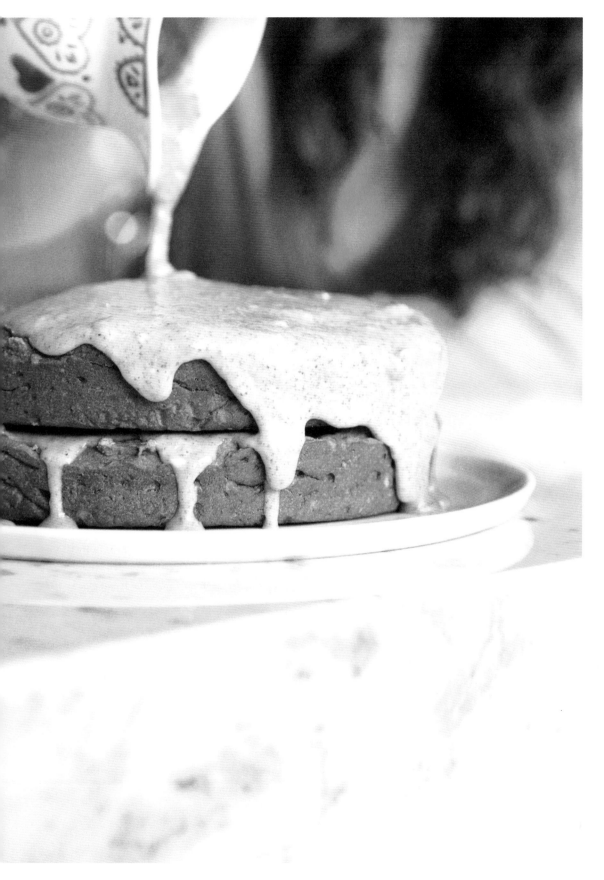

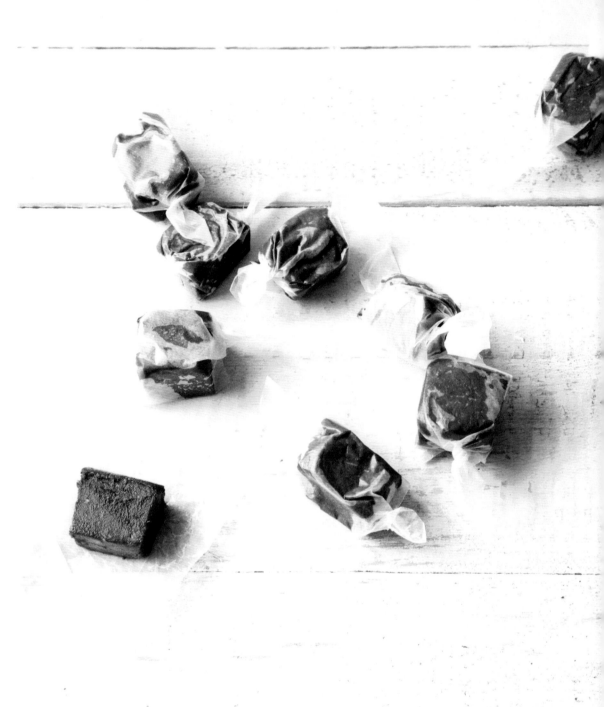

ALMOND BUTTER FUDGE

The first time I made this fudge my flatmates and I ate the whole batch within about 3 hours and then had to remake it the next day because we were craving it so much; it's that good – dangerously good even! Each bite is so gooey and chocolaty, it's crazy to think it's made from just four ingredients. The fudge is stored in the freezer, so you can make big batches of it at once, which means you always have something deliciously healthy to enjoy any time of the day.

makes about 20 fudge pieces
2 mugs Medjool dates (400g), pitted
10 tablespoons almond butter (recipe on page 24)
4 tablespoons coconut oil
3 tablespoons raw cacao powder

Place the dates in a saucepan with a little boiling water. Allow them to cook for 5 minutes, until they're really soft and all sticking together.

If there is any water left in the pan, then drain it and set the dates to one side to cool for a couple of minutes.

Place the almond butter, coconut oil and cacao powder in a food processor and add the dates in before blending for a minute or two, until a sticky paste forms.

Line a roughly 25cm baking dish with baking paper and pour the mix in before putting it into the freezer to set for at least 3 hours before serving.

Store in the freezer. When you want to enjoy a piece, take it out of the freezer and allow it to warm up for a few minutes before eating.

Top tip
Try adding chunks of nuts and raisins to this to change the texture and add more of a crunch.

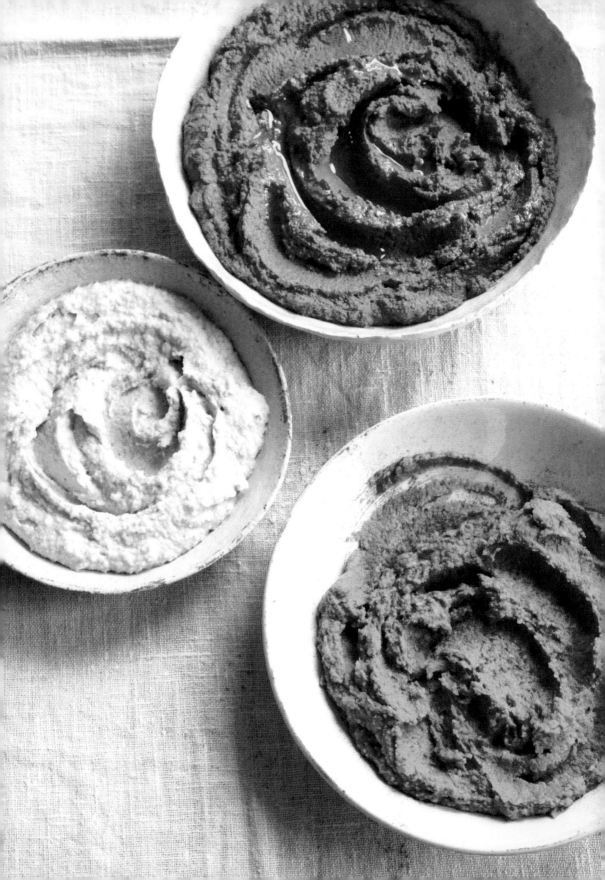

BEANS AND PULSES

nutritional powerhouses

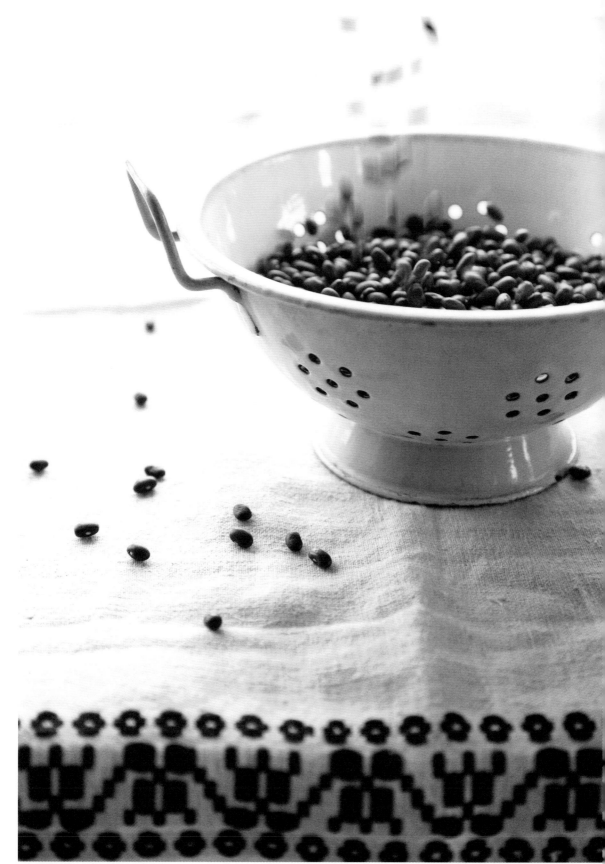

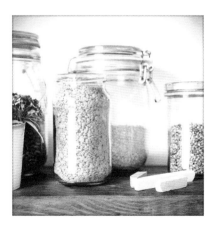

beans and pulses

Beans and pulses do have an unusual texture, which isn't to everyone's liking, and lots of people tend to shy away from them because of that. I used to fall into that category too, assuming that all pulses were like the beans you find in Heinz baked beans, i.e. slightly bland and mushy, until I started experimenting with them and realised that they were, in fact, totally awesome and I had been really missing out. It took me a while to start eating them, but once I started to really love plants, I thought I had to brave beans and pulses and I was converted so quickly! They really don't taste like Heinz baked beans at all, and the variety of different types of pulses means that there is bound to be one out there that you will love. The other thing is that not only do they taste really great, but they're really good for us too and they're incredibly inexpensive, so you can bulk up a meal very easily using a tin of beans.

The main reason that pulses are so important as part of a plant-based diet is that they're bursting with plant protein and fibre. They do contain a good selection of vitamins and minerals too, which is why some people claim that they're one of your five-a-day, but they don't really compare to fruits and veggies in this way, so I prefer to celebrate their incredible protein and dietary fibre content.

We need plant protein to sustain our energy levels all day, stop sugar cravings and fight off tiredness slumps, which in turn keeps our mood in a constant state of happiness. We need fibre for similar reasons. The more fibre something has, the slower its energy is released into your body. This helps to keep our blood sugar levels balanced, which in turn means that you'll stay energised and sated for longer, so you won't be reaching for a chocolate bar right after your meal – although you may still be dreaming of things like sweet potato brownies, simply because they are just so good! To give you some idea of how much fibre pulses contain, a small bowl of cooked lentils or black beans gives you around sixty per cent of your required intake of fibre – so they're pretty great things to eat if you want to look and feel amazing!

So what actually is a pulse? In short, it's an edible seed that grows in a pod. There are lots of different types of pulses available, the most common being lentils, chickpeas, black beans, cannellini beans, haricot beans and kidney beans, but even within these there are so many varieties. So I thought it would be helpful to give you a run-down of each of the main types, what they taste like and what I use them for, which you'll find below.

In terms of cooking pulses, you can either buy dried or tinned versions of everything. As a rule, dried pulses (excluding lentils) need to be soaked for four to six hours and then cooked before you can eat them, which can be a pain and does require a bit of advanced organisation. On the plus side, however, dried pulses are much cheaper than tinned ones and you know that no preservatives or sugar have been added to them. Tinned pulses are much quicker and easier to use, you just open the tin, drain and rinse the contents and then you can eat them immediately. Just be careful to read the ingredient list on the tin to make sure nothing else has been added to them. Beans are in season and available all year round too, which is awesome, so they're always easy to find and always taste good.

I keep my cupboards stocked with lots of tins of black beans, chickpeas, cannellini beans and lentils. Once these are open, they need to be stored in the fridge, but before that you can just leave them at room temperature. If you're keeping dried versions of the pulses, then you'll need to keep them in airtight containers, again at room temperature.

BLACK BEANS

Of all the beans, black beans are my favourite. I use them most days and really start to crave them when I don't have them. They have the best texture, slightly soft yet still nicely hearty. They have a strong taste too, which some people think is a bit like mushrooms, so they add a delicious savoury and earthy note to whatever you're making. My favourite thing to do with them is

to sauté them with a little garlic, miso paste and tomato purée – it's honestly so divine! I then normally mix them with precooked brown rice and mashed avocado for an awesome five-minute dinner when I don't have much time. They work really well with any grain though, which is how I normally use them. They're especially good in my Black and Kidney Bean Chilli with brown rice (page 114).

CHICKPEAS (GARBANZO BEANS)

I'm a little obsessed with chickpeas, not because they're that exciting on their own, but because they're the key ingredient in hummus. And I love hummus, a lot. In fact, I'll admit, it's a total addiction and I can't really go a day without it. It comes in so many delicious variations, my favourite of which I've included in this chapter – Classic, Beetroot, and Roasted Red Pepper and Paprika (page 102).

I love adding chickpeas to curries too. As they're that bit bigger than lentils they don't get lost, but add a delicious texture to each bite. They also have a great firm texture, which is amazing roasted. My Spicy Roasted Chickpeas (page 112) are really one of the best snacks ever. Like lentils, they're fibre bombs too, so they keep you energised for hours.

CANNELLINI BEANS

I have to be honest and admit that I don't find cannellini beans hugely exciting. They don't have a huge flavour like black beans or lentils, nor do they have a firm texture like chickpeas or kidney beans – they're much softer and mushier. That's not to say that they don't have their uses though – they really do, particularly for making soups (page 105). I always find that puréed veggie soups aren't filling enough on their own and I'm hungry an hour or so later, so I simply stir in puréed cannellini beans to my finished soup. This might sound a bit weird, but it really works magic in soups as it makes them much thicker and creamier, which is always amazing, whilst also making them much more satisfying and filling.

KIDNEY BEANS

Kidney beans really have a great texture. They taste similar to black beans, but they're more solid so they hold their shape better when they're cooked. You'll really taste the difference between the two in the Black and Kidney Bean Chilli recipe (page 114). This means that they cannot be blended as well as black beans into your grains, but stand out more on their own, which is really great in stews, chillies and curries. If you've always been a bit nervous of beans because of their 'mushy', Heinz baked beans-style texture, then these are a great bean to start experimenting with!

LENTILS

Lentils come in so many varieties; you have green lentils, brown lentils, puy lentils, red lentils, black lentils and yellow lentils. By and large I tend to use green, black or brown lentils, mainly because they're normally less expensive and easier to find in normal supermarkets. These three varieties also tend to retain their shape better while cooking, whilst the others can become slightly soft and mushy (lots of people like this though, so if you do, please feel free to replace with the red or yellow ones). The flavour is pretty much the same for all of them though.

To be honest I don't think they taste of a huge amount on their own, but what I do love about them is their lovely hearty texture and their slightly nutty taste. The best thing about them is that they really soak up the flavours of whatever they're cooked with so – if you follow my recipes – they end up tasting of a lot. I like to use lentils in salads, to make delicious dhals (page 119) or in my Bolognese (page 117).

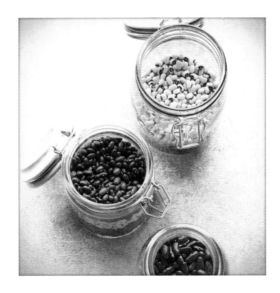

THREE TYPES OF HUMMUS

I could honestly live off hummus! I love that you can eat it with anything, from crudités to quinoa bowls, simple salads and, of course, spread over toast with some avocado. It adds a great protein boost to your meal too. Since I eat it so much, I like to vary the flavours, so I've shared my three favourites with you here: Classic, Beetroot, and Roasted Red Pepper and Paprika.

makes 1 large bowl

CLASSIC HUMMUS

2 x 400g tins of chickpeas, drained (or 450g drained chickpeas if you're soaking and boiling your own)
10 tablespoons olive oil
juice of 2 juicy lemons
2 heaped tablespoons tahini
3 cloves of garlic, peeled
2 teaspoons ground cumin
salt and pepper

Simply place all of the ingredients into a food processor with 3 tablespoons water and blend until smooth; it's really that easy! The stronger your food processor, the smoother and creamier the hummus will be.

Store it in an airtight container in the fridge for up to a week.

BEETROOT HUMMUS

1 quantity of classic hummus (recipe above)
1 small raw beetroot (150g), peeled and chopped

Place the hummus and beetroot in a food processor and blend until smooth and creamy.

ROASTED RED PEPPER AND PAPRIKA HUMMUS

2 large red peppers
1 quantity of classic hummus (recipe above)
½ jalapeño pepper (add more or less depending on how spicy you like it)
2 teaspoons paprika

Preheat the oven to 210°C (fan 190°C).

Start by slicing the red peppers into about eight long strips, discarding the seedy centre part. Place these strips on a baking tray and bake for 10 minutes until they begin to brown slightly.

Once the pepper has cooked and is starting to turn ever so slightly brown at the edges, remove from the oven and allow to cool for a couple of minutes.

Add the pepper to the food processor with the hummus, jalapeño pepper and paprika and blend until smooth.

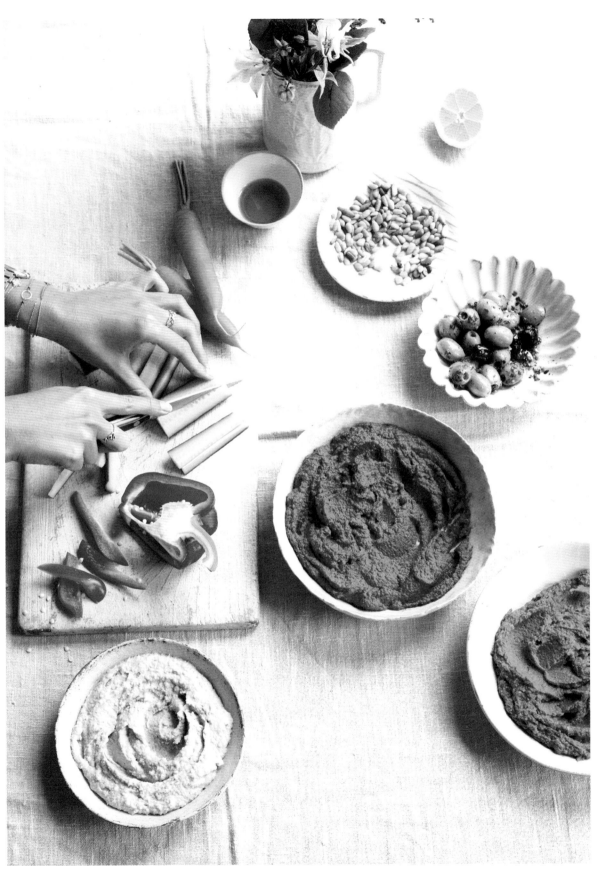

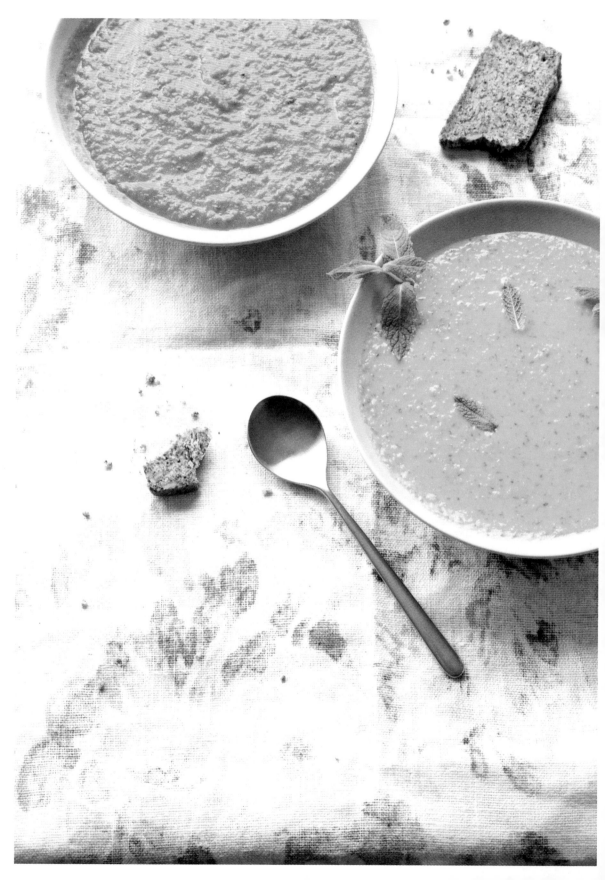

CANNELLINI SOUP TWO WAYS

Cannellini beans are the most wonderful soup ingredient. They make each mouthful extra thick and creamy, while also adding the protein you need to feel satisfied and energised after your bowl. Both of these soups are equally delicious and I'm sure you'll adore both. The pea and mint is also wonderful cold on a summer's day, while the roasted tomato and red pepper version is the best winter comfort food. I serve both with a side of my Superfood Crackers (page 82) or a few slices of Superfood Bread (page 80).

Serves 4

ROASTED TOMATO WITH RED PEPPER AND BASIL

16 large tomatoes

4 red peppers

4 tablespoons dried herbs (I like herbes de Provence, rosemary, thyme and oregano)

olive oil, for drizzling

2 large handfuls of fresh basil leaves

1 x 400g tin cannellini beans

4 tablespoons tomato purée

4 mugs stock or water (1.2 litres)

2 tablespoons tamari

salt and pepper

Preheat the oven to 190°C (fan 170°C).

Slice the tomatoes into about four pieces and the peppers into thick strips.

Place these on a baking tray with the dried herbs, salt and pepper and then drizzle everything with olive oil.

Bake for about 30 minutes.

Place the roasted tomato and pepper into a blender with the basil, beans, tomato purée, stock or water and the tamari and blend until smooth.

Finally, heat the soup in a pan for a few minutes, season to taste and then serve.

PEA AND MINT

5 mugs peas (750g)

3⅓ mugs easy veggie stock (1 litre) (recipe on page 27)

1 x 400g tin cannellini beans

12 sprigs of fresh mint

salt and pepper

Place the peas and stock in a large saucepan and begin to heat gently.

Cook until the peas begin to boil, which should take about 10 minutes.

Take off the heat and mix the peas and stock with the cannellini beans and the mint leaves (remove them from their sprigs) in a blender until the soup is smooth and creamy.

Finally, heat the soup in a pan for a few minutes, season to taste and then serve.

Top tip

Try sautéing some extra beans with a little garlic, olive oil, salt and pepper and stirring them into the soup once it's made for extra deliciousness.

CHICKPEA FLOUR WRAPS

These wraps are amazingly simple; they only take 5 minutes to throw together, so they're perfect if you're looking for something delicious with minimal time and effort. I love filling these with so much goodness, usually using either guacamole or hummus as the base, and then lots of rocket, red pepper slices, cucumber and lime juice.

makes 4 wraps

2 tablespoons ground flaxseed
1 mug chickpea (gram) flour (130g)
1 teaspoon dried mixed herbs
olive oil, for greasing
salt and pepper

Add all of the ingredients except the olive oil into a mixing bowl with ⅔ mug (200ml) water.

Use a whisk to mix it all together, ensuring that the batter is nice and smooth.

Leave the batter for about 5 minutes to let it thicken.

While the batter thickens, place a frying pan on a high heat and rub olive oil over the bottom of it using a piece of kitchen roll.

Pour a quarter of the batter into the pan and spread it as thinly as possible into a circle. After about 2 minutes or so, when the wrap is no longer translucent on the top, flip the wrap over and allow the other side to cook.

Do the same thing with each wrap, ensuring that you wipe olive oil over the pan each time before pouring batter in. The wraps can be served hot or cold. If serving hot, then keep warm while you cook the others.

Store any wraps that you don't eat straight away in the fridge in an airtight container.

Top tip

Make lots of these and take them to work instead of a sandwich. You can freeze batches of them too, so that you always have some ready to go.

FALAFELS

Falafels are so delicious as they're packed with so much flavour thanks to their amazing mix of spices, from garlic and apple purée to lemon, cumin, turmeric, tahini and coriander. I love serving them with a simple rocket salad dressed with olive oil and lime juice, a sprinkling of pomegranate seeds and then lots of Beetroot Hummus (page 102). They're also amazing served with my Quinoa Tabbouleh (page 46) and classic hummus for a Middle-Eastern-inspired meal.

Serves 4

handful of fresh coriander, finely chopped
2 cloves of garlic, peeled and crushed
juice of 2 lemons
2 tablespoons olive oil
2 tablespoons date syrup (you could also use
    honey – it must be a sticky sweetener)
2 tablespoons apple purée (recipe on page 19)
1 tablespoon ground cumin
1 tablespoon ground turmeric
1 tablespoon tahini
800g tinned chickpeas, drained
½ mug pine nuts (65g)
sprinkling of brown rice or chickpea flour
salt and pepper

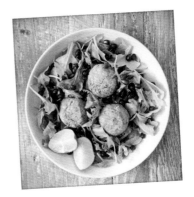

Preheat the oven to 200°C (fan 180°C).

Add all the ingredients, except the chickpeas, pine nuts, brown rice or chickpea flour, to a food processor. Blend until everything is mixed well, but the texture is still a little chunky and not totally smooth.

Place the chickpeas and pine nuts in the food processor and blend for about 20 seconds until they are broken up, but haven't totally disintegrated into hummus.

Roll the mixture into about twelve balls using your hands and place these in the fridge for about 30 minutes to set.

Once set, remove them from the fridge, coat them in brown rice or chickpea flour and bake them for 45 minutes until the outside is nice and crispy.

Top tip
These can be served hot or cold, so in the winter eat them as a warming, nourishing food with sautéed spinach and in the summer enjoy them with salad.

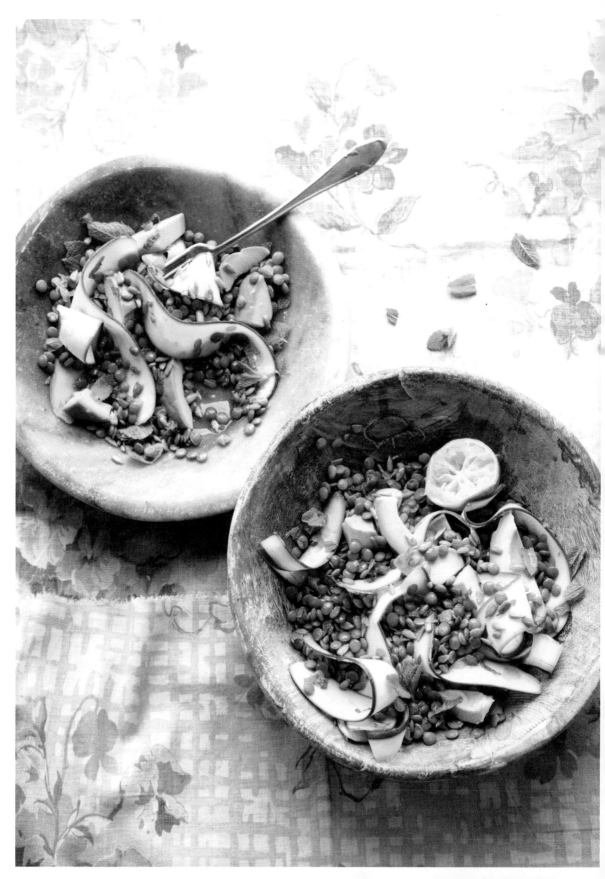

LENTIL, COURGETTE AND MINT SALAD

I taught this salad in my cooking classes last summer and everyone loved it. It's so fresh and summery with a delicious array of simple flavours. The thin strips of courgette melt against the creamy chunks of avocado, while the lentils add a hearty, satisfying element and the mint leaves and lime juice make it all taste so fresh. I love sprinkling sunflower seeds over the top for a little crunch too! This is amazing served a side of steamed or sautéed green veggies.

Serves 4

½ mug green lentils (100g)
3 medium courgettes
2 handfuls of fresh mint
2 avocados
4 tablespoons olive oil
juice of 4 limes
large handful of sunflower seeds

Place the lentils in boiling water and allow them to boil for 10 minutes, then let them simmer for about 30 minutes until they're soft, but not mushy. If there's any water left in the pan, drain and then allow the lentils to cool.

While the lentils cool, peel the courgettes into thin strips using a potato peeler. Pull the mint leaves off the stems and roughly chop them into pieces. Slice the avocado into bite-sized chunks.

Place the cooled lentils, courgette strips, avocado and mint in a bowl and drizzle over the olive oil and lime juice. Mix well before sprinkling the sunflower seeds on the top.

Top tip

Try adding a variety of other ingredients to this salad to keep it interesting. I love adding pomegranate seeds, toasted cashew nuts, bean sprouts and thinly sliced mushrooms when I'm after something a little different.

'Your recipes have completely changed my life. I was diagnosed with M.E. nearly 3 years ago. A friend showed me your website and I thought I'd give it a go. Within a week I was jumping out of bed, skipping to work and going for a run every night. This was completely unheard of. Before, I had struggled to get out of bed, meaning a full-time job was a distant dream and I had to work part-time, never mind exercising! So all I can say is a massive thank you and I hope your book helps others as much as you have helped me!'
– Hannah

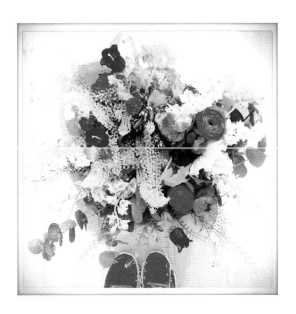

BAKED BEANS

I shared a photo of this dish on my Instagram and I've had people ask me almost every day when I'm going to be sharing the recipe – so here it is at last! I never used to like Heinz baked beans, but these are so delicious it's impossible not to love them. When I first created the recipe, I loved them so much that I ate them almost every day for at least a month! They taste amazing for brunch with a slice of my Giant Hash Browns (page 130), but they're equally delicious for lunch or dinner with my Marinated Kale Salad (page 153) or with a simple side of brown rice.

Serves 4

250g tinned haricot beans, drained

2 cloves of garlic, peeled and crushed

2 x 400g tins chopped tomatoes

2 tablespoons date syrup

1 tube tomato purée (200g)

salt and pepper

First peel and crush the garlic. Place the crushed garlic in a large saucepan with the tins of chopped tomatoes and the date syrup.

Allow the mixture to boil and then cook over a low heat for about 30 minutes.

At this point, add the tomato purée and the beans and cook with the sauce for another 10 minutes or so until everything is really hot and the sauce is nice and thick and not overly runny. Season with the salt and pepper to taste.

SPICY ROASTED CHICKPEAS

These spicy roasted chickpeas make the best snack as they're full of flavour, but they're also awesome sprinkled onto salads to create extra texture or used instead of croutons in soup. I particularly love them in my Warm Wild Rice Salad (page 40) and on my Roasted Tomato with Red Pepper and Basil Soup (page 105).

Makes 1 large jar

500g tinned chickpeas

1 tablespoon paprika

1 tablespoon ground cumin

2 teaspoons chilli flakes (add more if you like spice)

2 tablespoons maple syrup

juice of 1 lemon

olive oil

salt and pepper

Preheat the oven to 200°C (fan 180°C).

Drain the chickpeas and place them on a large baking tray.

Sprinkle the paprika, cumin, chilli flakes and salt and pepper onto them and then drizzle over the maple syrup, lemon juice and some olive oil, stirring well to ensure that everything is evenly coated.

Bake for about 45 minutes, until the chickpeas are nice and crunchy.

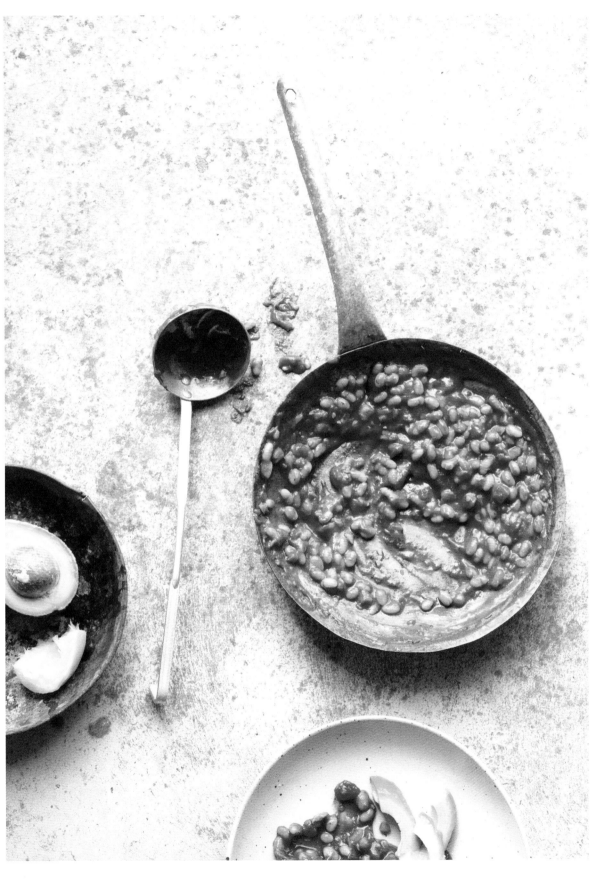

BLACK AND KIDNEY BEAN CHILLI

This is one of the simplest and most nourishing recipes in the book. It only takes 10 minutes to put together and it's wonderfully filling and comforting. It's one of my go-to meals all winter. It's a great dish to make if you're feeding lots of people too as it's no more complicated to make for twelve then it is for two. It requires almost no chopping, so you won't be in the kitchen for hours!

Serves 4

2 carrots, grated

2 cloves of garlic, peeled and crushed

600g passata

50g tomato purée

2 x 400g tins black beans

1 x 400g tin red kidney beans

1 jalapeño pepper, deseeded and finely chopped

1 teaspoon chilli flakes (add more if you like it extra spicy)

brown rice, to serve

salt and pepper

Place the carrot and garlic into a large saucepan.

Add the passata, tomato purée, both the beans, jalapeño pepper and the chilli flakes to the saucepan along with some salt and pepper, to taste.

Cook the chilli for about 10 minutes, stirring it well, until it's lovely and warm and everything's nicely mixed together.

Pour the chilli over brown rice and enjoy.

Top tip

Make extra batches of this and freeze them as it makes a delicious, filling meal when you don't have time to prepare anything.

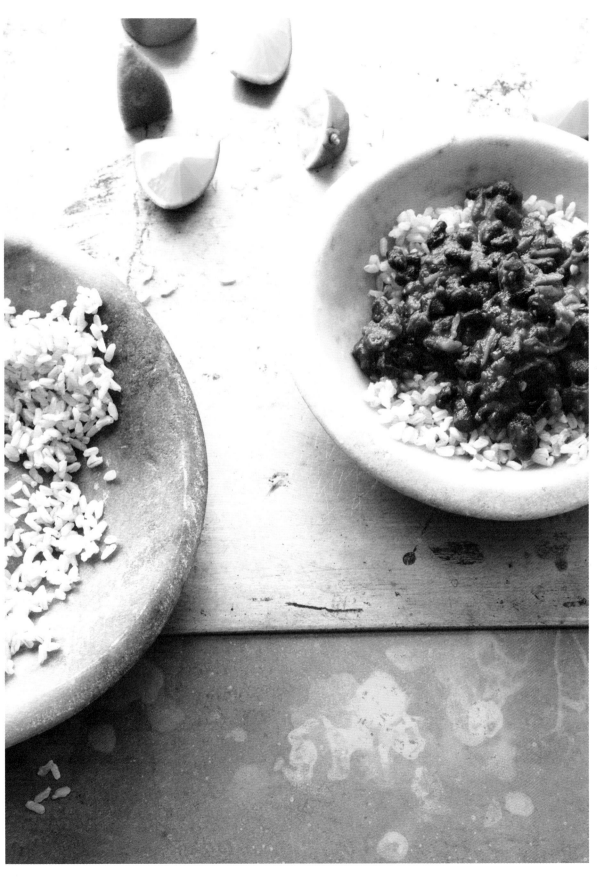

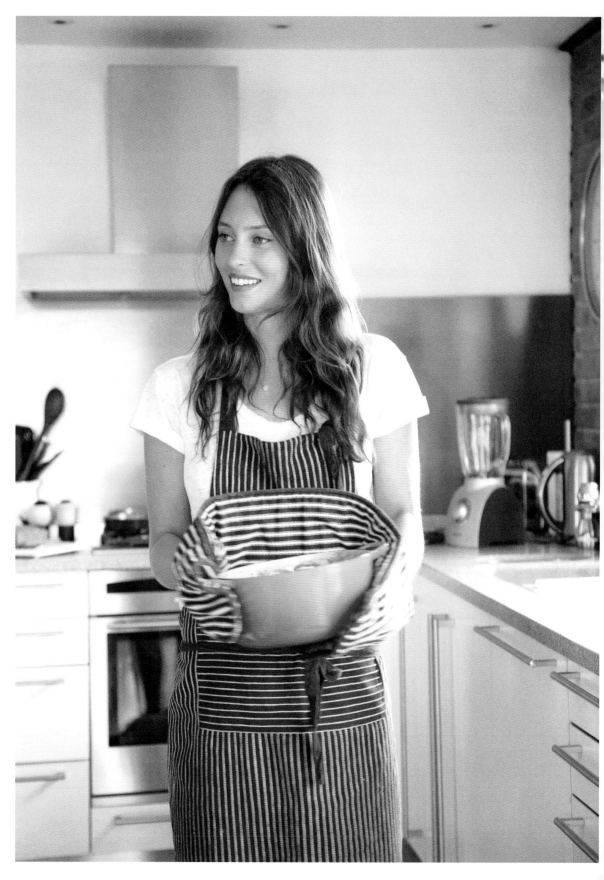

LENTIL BOLOGNESE

I had a big group of girlfriends taste-test this recipe and they all went back for thirds, proclaiming that this was so much better than beef bolognese, so I knew the recipe had to go in the book! Like the Lentil and Butternut Squash Dhal (page 119) and the Black and Kidney Bean Chilli (page 114), this bolognese is an incredibly easy recipe to make both for yourself and for big groups as there's so little preparation involved in it; plus the ingredients are easy to find anywhere and they're all really inexpensive.

Serves 4

3 large carrots (450g)
175g sun-dried tomatoes
3 cloves of garlic, peeled and crushed
2 x 400g tins chopped tomatoes
2 tubes of tomato purée (400g)
2½ mugs green lentils (500g)
500g gluten-free pasta
salt and pepper

Start by peeling and grating the carrots using the coarse side of your grater. Chop the sun-dried tomatoes into small pieces.

Add the grated carrot, chopped sun-dried tomatoes and crushed garlic to a large saucepan with the tins of chopped tomatoes, tomato purée, lentils and 1½ mugs (450ml) boiling water.

Stir everything together and then allow the mixture to simmer for 45 minutes to an hour, stirring it every now and again as it cooks.

Once it's almost ready, cook the pasta until al dente, drain it and mix it into the bolognese. Serve with pasta.

Top tip
You can try adding some kidney beans to this at the end to give it an even chunkier texture and an extra boost of protein.

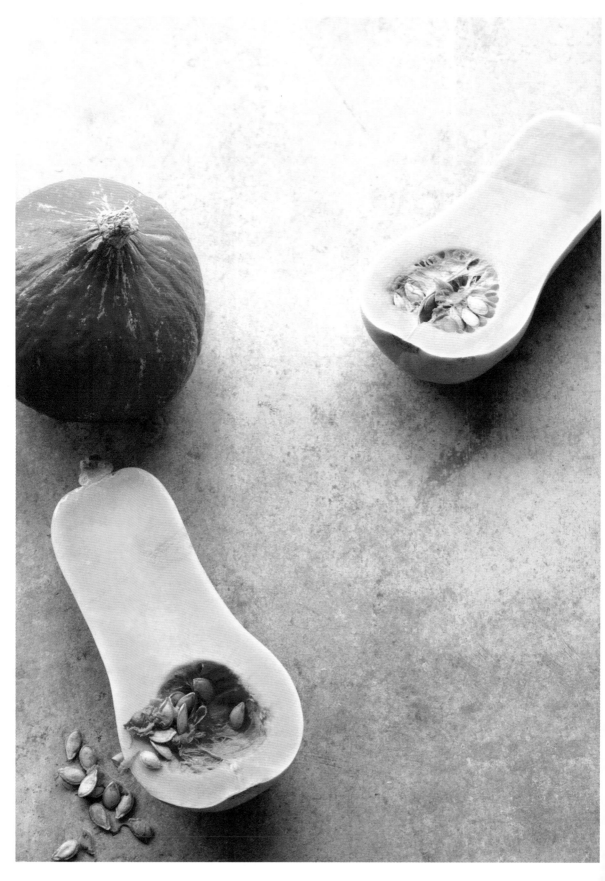

LENTIL AND BUTTERNUT SQUASH DHAL

This is a slightly untraditional dhal as it uses green lentils instead of red lentils, but I prefer the slightly hearty texture that they create – I'm not the biggest fan of totally mushy lentils. Saying that, you can absolutely swap them around; you'll just need to cook them for a slightly shorter amount of time. I love this served over a plate of warm brown rice. It's a fantastically inexpensive meal, and like the Black and Kidney Bean Chilli (page 114), it's really to easy to make this for lots of people with minimal stress!

Serves 4

4 cloves of garlic, peeled and crushed
2-3cm piece of fresh ginger, peeled and grated
1 tablespoon olive oil
1 mug green lentils (200g)
1 large butternut squash (1kg)
2 tablespoons ground cumin
2 tablespoons ground turmeric
2 tablespoons tomato purée
brown rice, to serve
salt and pepper

Place the crushed garlic and grated ginger in a frying pan with the olive oil and fry for a couple of minutes. During this time, boil the kettle.

Add the lentils to a large saucepan with the ginger and garlic and cover them with 2 mugs (500ml) boiling water. Allow the pan to start simmering.

Peel and cut the squash into small bite-sized pieces and add these to the lentils with the cumin, turmeric, tomato purée, salt and pepper.

Put the lid on the pan and leave it to simmer for about 40 minutes, at which point the lentils and the squash should be soft. You may need to add a little more water during this time.

Then serve with brown rice.

Top tip

You can swap the butternut squash for any other veggie you like; aubergine and sweet potato are my other two favourites.

COCONUT THAI CURRY WITH CHICKPEAS

This Coconut Thai Curry was the first recipe I did for this book and it's still one of my favourites! The coconut milk makes it wonderfully creamy, while the ginger, chilli flakes, coriander and miso add a fantastic array of different flavours. The chickpeas make it really hearty too, so it's amazingly filling. I love it served with brown rice, but it's delicious with buckwheat too or brown rice pasta. It keeps really well, so you can make extra portions of it to store in the fridge to fuel you through the week.

Serves 4

2 x 400ml tins coconut milk
2 x 400g tins tomatoes
2-3cm piece of fresh ginger, peeled and grated
1-2 teaspoons chilli flakes
1 large butternut squash (1kg)
2 medium aubergines (600g)
handful of fresh coriander, finely chopped
1 x 400g tin chickpeas, drained
3 teaspoons brown miso paste
brown rice, to serve
salt and pepper

Preheat the oven to 200°C (fan 180°C).

Put the coconut milk, tinned tomatoes, grated ginger and chilli into a large saucepan with a sprinkling of salt and pepper and allow it to heat until boiling.

As it heats up, peel the squash and cut both the squash and the aubergines into bite-sized pieces. Add these to the coconut and tomato in the pan.

Allow the mixture to cook for about 30 minutes in the oven, at which point add the coriander and chickpeas to the pan with the miso and place the pan back in the oven for 30 minutes. It's ready when the squash is soft.

Serve the coconut curry with the brown rice. Store any leftovers in an airtight container in the fridge or freezer.

Top tip

If you don't like chickpeas, you can leave these out. You can also substitute any of the veggies for other ones you have in the house; cauliflower, courgettes and sweet potatoes are all delicious.

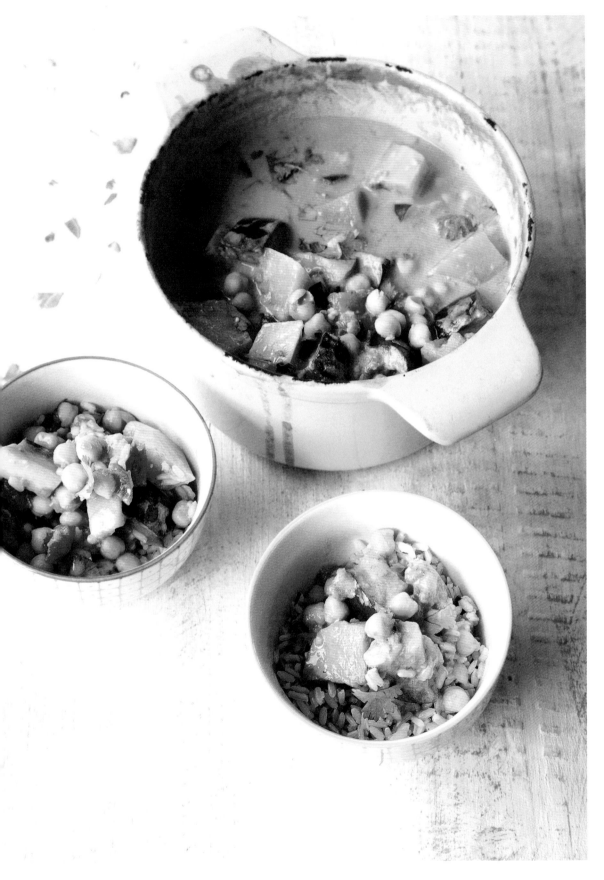

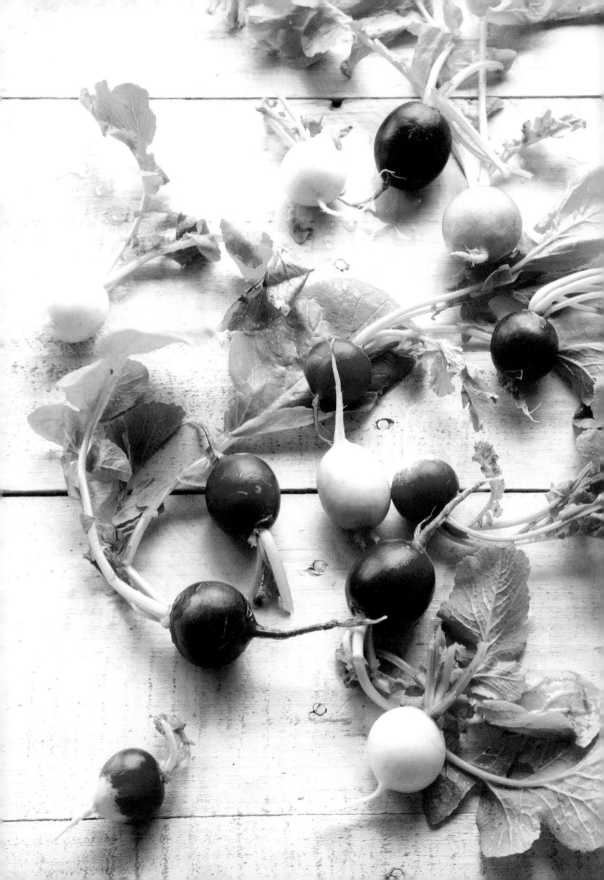

EASY ROAST VEGGIES

CLASSIC MASHED POTATO

GIANT HASH BROWN

TEN-MINUTE TOMATO PASTA

SWEET POTATO WEDGES

PERFECT ROAST POTATOES

SPICY SALSA

PAN CON TOMATE

CUCUMBER AND AVOCADO ROLLS

CARROT, ORANGE AND CASHEW SALAD

BEETROOT CARPACCIO

VEGETABLES

more exciting than you may think

CLASSIC STIR-FRY

ROASTED SQUASH, OLIVE, AVOCADO AND ROCKET SALAD

BROCCOLI AND AVOCADO SALAD

STUFFED CHESTNUT MUSHROOMS

MARINATED KALE SALAD

WARM WINTER SALAD

VEGGIE LASAGNE

CAULIFLOWER AND POTATO CURRY

BROCCOLI WITH A TAHINI DRESSING

CLASSIC GUACAMOLE

COURGETTE NOODLES WITH AVOCADO PESTO

SWEET POTATO PANCAKES

BEETROOT CHOCOLATE CAKE WITH COCONUT FROSTING

SWEET POTATO BROWNIES

EASY AVOCADO CHOCOLATE MOUSSE

CLASSIC CARROT CAKE WITH CARAMEL FROSTING

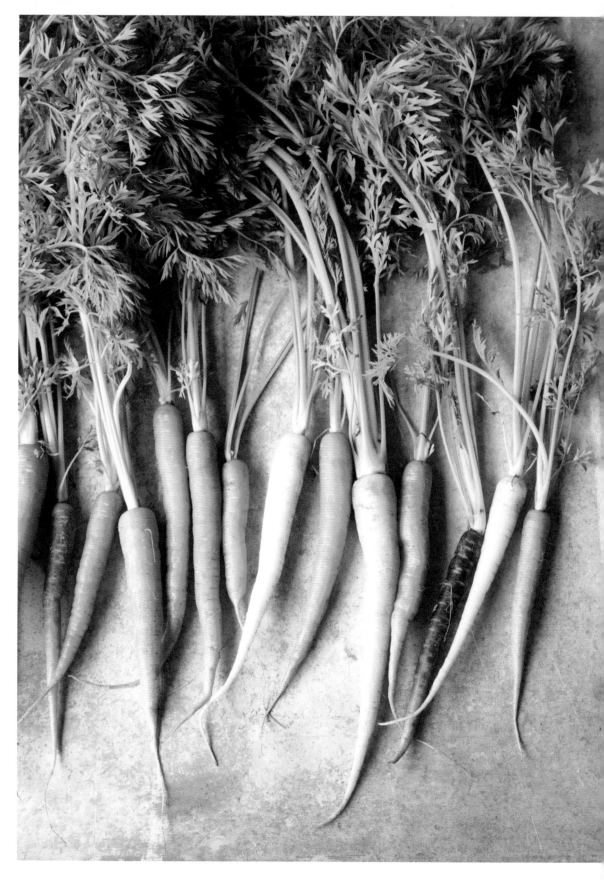

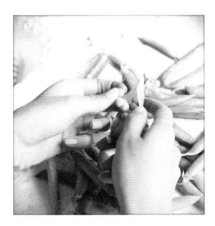

vegetables

I think it's fair to say that traditionally vegetables have always been the side dish and generally speaking they're an afterthought that most people don't get too excited about. Growing up in a 'meat and two veg' country like the UK, I thought like this too, until I started experimenting with them and realised that you can actually make magic happen with vegetables – it's all about how they're cooked and what they're paired with.

Normally vegetables are boiled or steamed, sometimes microwaved, and maybe roasted, but I find that rarely are they done in a way that makes them truly delicious and the heart of a meal. We often feel obliged to eat them because we know we should, but we don't fall head over heels in love with them and most people certainly don't dream of broccoli! I've been given plates of totally plain steamed veggies before in restaurants and even I – the biggest veggie lover around – didn't really enjoy my meal, so I do understand that most people find it hard to get that excited about them. I promise though that once you learn how to take advantage of their incredible natural flavours and let me help you discover how to cook them

in interesting ways, you'll start to adore them. As you discover new ways to cook them, you'll want vegetables to be the biggest part of your meal, and the delicious discoveries that you make will mean that you'll naturally want to start eating more of them. Pretty soon they'll no longer feel like an obligation but something you really want to eat! Once you feel this way about your veggies, healthy eating and living become a natural part of your life, which is awesome. This is what happened to me and it changed both my health and my life in the best way!

So how do we make them delicious? We need to get creative! It's all about seasoning them with fresh herbs and wonderful spices and adding fantastic sauces, rich dressings and creamy dips. I want to introduce you to delicious dishes like the Warm Winter Salad (page 154), Cucumber and Avocado Rolls (page 136), thinly sliced strips of Beetroot Carpaccio (page 140) or tamari-smothered Kale Salad with Pomegranate (page 153).

How good does that all sound? There really are so many ways that you can cook your veggies and so many ways that you can spice and marinate them, all of which will give you a totally different perspective on things that always seemed pretty mundane before. It may seem like more work to begin with as you start to focus on giving your veggies love and attention, but after a few weeks it becomes totally natural and won't seem any more time-consuming than cooking anything else – it's just a different mindset.

The next part might sound basic, but it's actually really important to learn about the different ways of cooking your veggies and when to use each way, because that really makes a huge difference to what you're making.

STEAMING

I normally steam my veggies if I want them to be very soft and squishy. Steaming doesn't accentuate the flavour especially, but it does tend to make the veggies soft, so it's easy to purée them and get a smooth, creamy texture to make things like risottos, simple purées for sweet recipes or dips. Steaming is also awesome as it allows almost all the goodness of the vegetables to be retained, so it's a very nutritious way to cook. I tend to avoid steaming if I'm eating my veggies on their own, as the end taste isn't overly exciting. You also can't season them as they cook, so it's harder to create amazing flavours at the end.

ROASTING

Roasting is the best way to draw the flavour out of your veg and is my favourite way to add extra flavour while cooking. It also gives vegetables a crispy outside, while the inside tends to stay nicely tender – so there is a great texture contrast going on in each bite. I find roasting works with almost every veg, but I especially love it with heartier veggies, things like sweet potatoes, carrots, parsnips, squash, carrots, aubergines and beetroots, and if I'm eating any of these on their own, I always make them this way. The only things I would avoid really are your greens and leafy veggies – cucumber, celery, spinach and green beans don't roast so well.

Roasting is my favourite way to experiment with spices too. You can add things like cumin, turmeric, paprika and cinnamon right at the beginning so that the veggies really soak up all the flavours and aromas while they cook. This creates a much stronger flavour than if the spices were added at the end, while also helping to accentuate the natural flavours of whatever you're cooking.

SAUTÉING

Sautéing is fantastic if you're after something speedy. You can sauté an amazing mixture of things like broccoli, courgettes, peppers and baby corn in less than 10 minutes. As with roasting, it's easy to season your veggies when you cook this way and you can throw in any number of sauces or pestos too to spice things up. I love adding some of my Brazil Nut and Rocket Pesto (page 86) or some finely chopped tomatoes and tomato purée to make a tomato sauce, for instance. You have to be a little more careful here not to burn things and your veggies won't be quite as flavoursome as if they were roasted, but it's a very convenient way to cook and it's much more delicious than steaming or boiling.

BOILING

Boiling is the only method that I tend to avoid, unless I'm cooking potatoes or frozen peas. It's quite damaging to the nutrient levels of your veggies and it really doesn't do much for their flavour. Steaming vegetables is a much better option as it takes just the same amount of time, but their goodness is retained. Boiling veggies just makes them very bland and it will take a lot more work to get them tasting delicious at the end. Whatever you add will just sit on top of your veggies, rather than be absorbed into them, in the way that roasting or sautéing does.

MICROWAVING

I should quickly say that I don't own a microwave and never use one. They're very damaging to the nutrient levels of your food and they don't bring out any flavour. It's much better to use any of the other methods I've discussed rather than microwave.

THE BEST ADDITIONS TO MAKE THEM DELICIOUS

I've talked a lot about my pantry staples in the first chapter, so I won't go into too much detail here on what each ingredient does, but these are the things that I would reach for to spice up my veggies:

Freshly squeezed lemon, lime or apple cider vinegar for a tangy edge. I normally add one of the three to my sautéed veg and if I steam something, I always add one of them at the end to liven up the dish.

Tamari for a rich, salty flavour. It's great in a lot of sauces and I almost always add it to my veggies when sautéing so that they can soak it up as they cook.

Tahini just tastes good with everything, as it makes anything deliciously creamy. I add this at the end of the cooking process and often drizzle it over my roasted veg once they've finished cooking or stir a spoonful into my sautéed veg towards the end to make a sort of sauce.

Cinnamon is my favourite spice. I love using it when I roast things to add a subtle sweetness to the dish. It works best with root veggies, as they are already a little sweet, so things like sweet potatoes, carrots and beets.

Paprika is another incredible spice; it's made from grinding dried peppers and, like cinnamon, it's slightly sweet. It tastes amazing in almost everything, especially anything with chilli as it really complements the spiciness.

Cumin is the spice used in hummus. It's delicious, but very strong and more savoury than paprika or cinnamon. It comes either as seeds or ground into a powder, both of which are great.

I normally use the powder, as it's easier to spread over your veggies so that they're all seasoned. I use it most in curries.

Turmeric is totally magical; it's one of the most healing things around as it's so anti-inflammatory. It's an Indian spice that's part of the ginger family. A classic curry ingredient, it tastes slightly warm, with a somewhat bitter, peppery flavour. It's delicious stirred into buckwheat dishes, mixed into salad dressings or used in curries.

Mixed herbs are such an important addition to any kitchen, and it's so worth investing in some good ones. I love herbes de Provence as it mixes together all my favourite herbs, but you can also just use a pinch of dried oregano, basil, thyme and rosemary and make your own mixed herbs. I use these on absolutely everything to add instant flavour.

Chilli flakes are another easy addition to anything to enhance the taste of whatever you're cooking and create a deeper range of flavours.

Fresh basil leaves are an amazing option, although unlike all the other ingredients these need to be bought fresh and can't be kept as a pantry staple. I try to keep a basil plant in my kitchen though so that I always have access to the leaves, which smell gorgeous. Basil is especially delicious with anything tomato-based, and can be used cooked or raw.

Fresh coriander is my second go-to fresh herb. It's more bitter than basil and has been described as having a taste similar to citrus peel. I'm not sure that it's the perfect description, but it gives you an idea of the sort of taste it has.

I have included all my favourite veggie recipes here. Hopefully you're now inspired to get started!

EASY ROAST VEGGIES

Roast veggies are one of the most delicious things in the world, especially if you season them well. These ones are baked with lots of paprika, thyme and rosemary, which makes them taste incredible. They're the perfect accompaniment to any meal; I love serving them with my Warm Wild Rice Salad (page 40), my Marinated Kale Salad (page 153) and my Stuffed Chestnut Mushrooms (page 150), although they work equally well as a meal on their own with a simple side of Hummus (page 102) for a protein boost. These last really well in the fridge too, so you can make big batches and take them to work with you for lunch for a few days.

Serves 4

1 large butternut squash
6 carrots
3 small sweet potatoes
olive oil
1 tablespoon dried mixed herbs
2 tablespoons paprika
big handful of fresh thyme
big handful of fresh rosemary
salt and pepper

Preheat the oven to 200°C (fan 180°C).

Peel the butternut squash and carrots (the sweet potato doesn't need to be peeled). Then cut all three veggies into similar-sized chunks – they want to be just bigger than bite-sized.

Place them on a large baking tray, drizzling with a generous amount of olive oil.

Sprinkle the mixed herbs, paprika and salt and pepper on the veggies and mix them in well so that they're all evenly coated, then place the leaves of the fresh herbs on top of all the vegetables.

Place the tray in the oven and allow the veggies to cook for about an hour, until they're all nice and soft. You'll need to stir them once or twice during this time to make sure that they cook evenly.

Top tip

Make sure that the veggies don't all sit on top of each other when they bake, as this will stop them from cooking properly. Use either one large baking tray or a couple of smaller ones to avoid this.

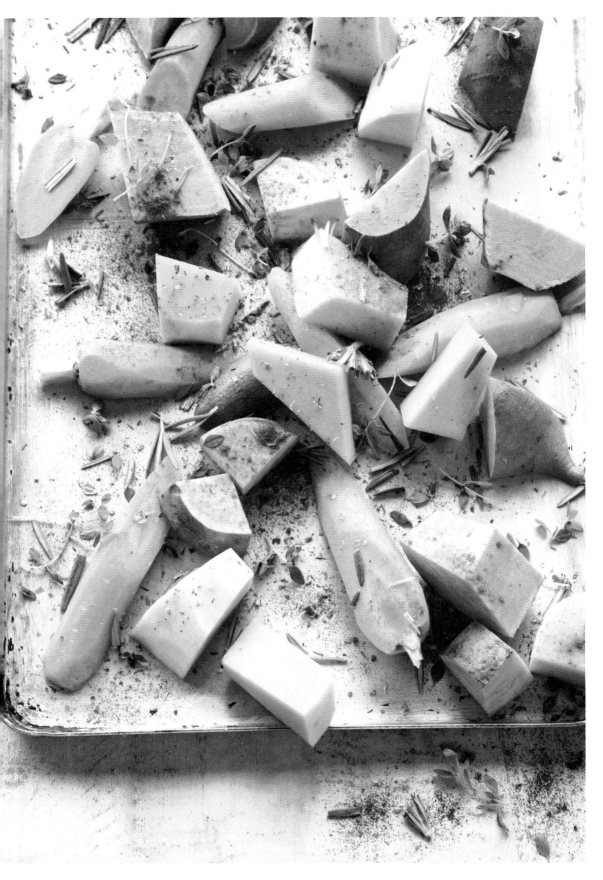

CLASSIC MASHED POTATO

I know dairy-free mashed potato sounds a little strange as the traditional recipe revolves around a mixture of butter and milk with a little cream, but trust me on this one, it really works without them – in fact I actually think it's more delicious.

Serves 4

10 medium potatoes (1.25kg)
½ mug olive oil (150ml)
1 tablespoon mustard seeds
salt and pepper

Peel the potatoes and chop them in half.

Place them in a pan and cover them in cold water, then begin cooking for about 40 minutes until you can easily put a knife through a potato.

Mash them until they fall apart and then add the olive oil, mustard seeds, salt and pepper and mash again until smooth and creamy.

GIANT HASH BROWN

Can you think of anything more delicious than a giant, super-crispy hash brown served with mashed avocado, garlicky tomatoes and home-made Baked Beans (page 112)? I really can't – it's the best brunch ever. The great thing is that the hash browns are so easy to make too and require very few ingredients, so you can whip them up any time!

Serves 4

5 medium potatoes (750g)
4 tablespoons brown rice flour
5 tablespoons apple purée
   (recipe on page 19)
olive oil
salt and pepper

Peel and grate the potatoes.

Wrap a clean tea towel around the grated potato and squeeze all the excess water from the potatoes using your hands into a bowl.

Discard the water and mix the dry grated potato into a clean bowl with the flour, apple purée, salt and pepper until everything is nice and sticky.

Cover the bottom of a large frying pan with olive oil and allow it to heat up for a couple of minutes.

Once the pan is nice and hot, add the potato mix to it, evenly covering the whole pan.

Turn the heat down to a medium setting and allow it to cook for 10 minutes before flipping.

To flip, place a plate on top of the pan and then turn the pan upside down so the hash brown stays on the plate. Place the uncooked side back on the pan and cook for another 10 minutes, until both sides are nicely browned.

Cut the giant hash brown into slices to serve.

TEN-MINUTE TOMATO PASTA

This pasta is the best thing to make when you're feeling lazy and have almost nothing in your fridge as the only fresh ingredient you need are tomatoes. It's such a warming, nourishing bowl too – the perfect comfort food! It requires very little chopping, which is always great. I eat this a lot when I'm home on my own in the evening.

Serves 4

600g pasta (I use brown rice pasta)
500g cherry tomatoes
2 x 400g tins tomatoes
4 tablespoons tomato purée
6 tablespoons apple cider vinegar
2 tablespoons tamari
2 x 400g tins black beans
optional: 1 bag of spinach
olive oil
salt and pepper

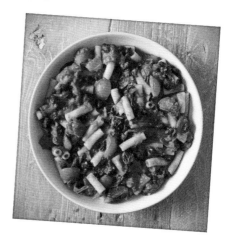

Cook the pasta. While the pasta cooks, make the sauce.

Start by chopping the cherry tomatoes into quarters, then place the chopped tomatoes into a large saucepan with the tinned tomatoes, tomato purée, apple cider vinegar and tamari, plus salt and pepper. Allow them to simmer into a sauce for about 5 minutes.

Open the tins of beans, rinse and drain them before stirring them into the sauce along with the spinach, if you're using it.

Once the pasta is ready, stir the sauce in and drizzle the olive oil over the top.

Top tip

Try adding any veggies that you have in your fridge to this pasta – things like grated carrot, slices of courgettes and sautéed mushrooms. It's a great way to use up any leftover ingredients.

SWEET POTATO WEDGES

These sweet potato wedges are one of my most loved recipes from the blog and one of my personal favourites too. I've made them hundreds of times and they're always so popular. I serve these as a side dish with just about everything, but I especially love them dunked into my Classic Guacamole (page 159).

Serves 4

3 large sweet potatoes
olive oil
1 heaped tablespoon ground
   cinnamon
1 heaped tablespoon paprika
dozen sprigs of fresh rosemary
salt

Preheat the oven to 200°C (fan 180°C).

Slice the sweet potatoes into thick wedges. Place these on a baking tray and drizzle a generous amount of olive oil over them. Then sprinkle the cinnamon, paprika and salt over them and stir well so that all the potatoes are covered with seasoning.

Lay the sprigs of rosemary on top of the potatoes. Finally, bake them for about an hour, turning them over once or twice during this time. You want them to cook until they're perfectly soft and tender.

PERFECT ROAST POTATOES

There's something so comforting and warming about roast potatoes. I really think they're one of the best pick-me-up foods when you're having a bad day – kind of like an edible hug! These potatoes are seasoned with fresh sprigs of rosemary and thyme so that the herbs can sink into the potatoes as they roast, ensuring that every bite has maximum flavour! I love serving them with my Quinoa and Turmeric Fritters (page 50) and they're also delicious chopped up and stirred into soup instead of croutons.

Serves 4

about 12 medium potatoes
   (1.5kg) (I like Maris Piper
   potatoes)
olive oil
dozen sprigs of fresh thyme
dozen sprigs of fresh rosemary
salt and pepper

Preheat the oven to 200°C (fan 180°C).

Peel the potatoes, then slice them in half.

Place the potatoes in a saucepan of cold water and bring them to the boil.

Once they've reached the boil, let them cook for a couple of minutes before removing them from the heat and draining them.

Next, place them in a baking tray with a generous amount of olive oil, salt and pepper and place the herbs on top of them.

Leave them to cook for about an hour, turning them once or twice during this time to ensure they cook evenly.

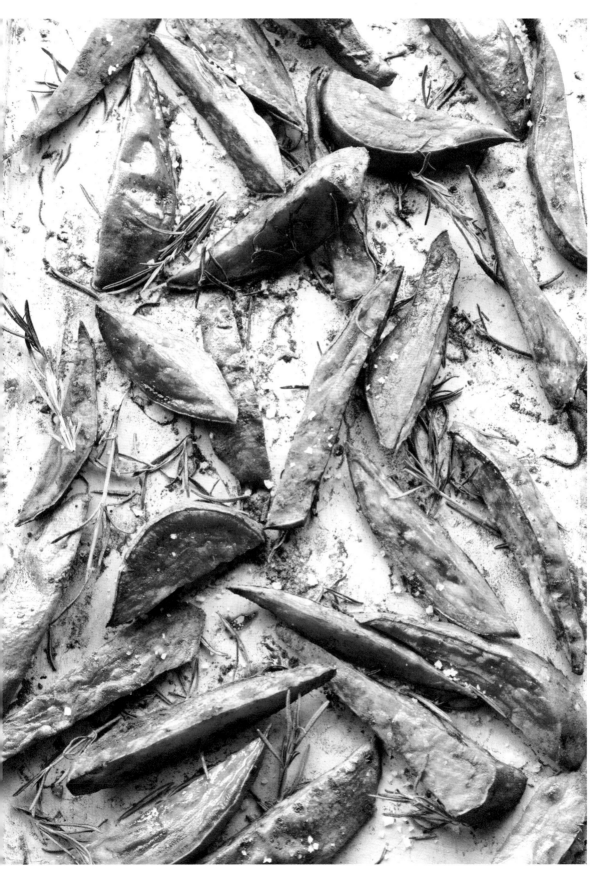

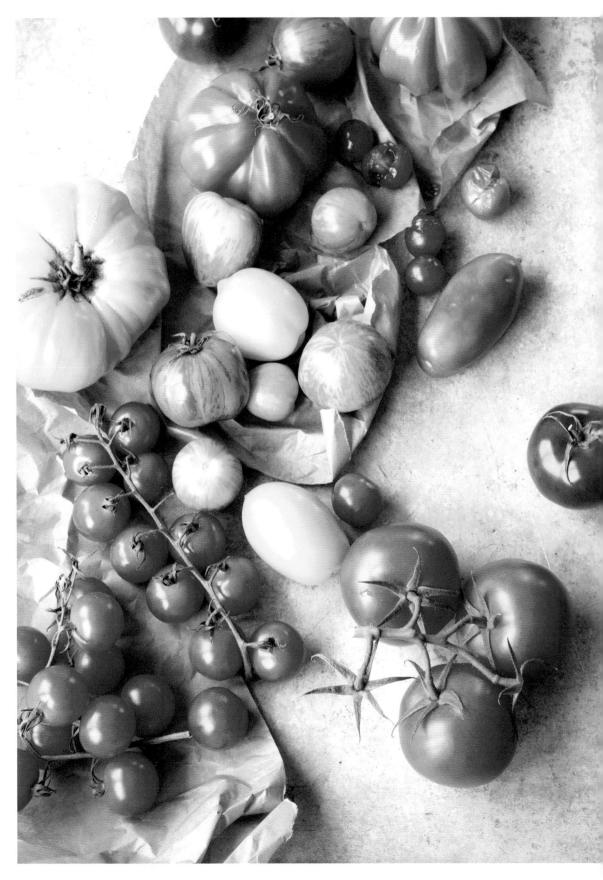

SPICY SALSA

Salsa is another really easy dish that automatically adds flavour to a meal. Plus it's a very inexpensive dish. I love piling lots of salsa and guacamole into a Chickpea Flour Wrap (page 106) with some sweetcorn, rocket leaves and black beans: it makes the perfect summer meal.

makes 1 bowl

4 tomatoes
1 jalapeño pepper
handful of fresh coriander
juice of 1 lime
3 tablespoons olive oil
sprinkling of chilli flakes
salt and pepper

Slice the tomatoes really finely into very small cubes.

Slice the jalapeño in half, remove all the seeds, then dice.

Remove the coriander leaves from the stem, then chop the leaves finely (I find it easiest to put the coriander in a mug and chop it with scissors).

Place the chopped tomatoes, jalapeño and coriander into a bowl, then squeeze the lime juice in and add the olive oil, salt, chilli flakes and pepper.

Stir well before serving.

PAN CON TOMATE

This is my brother's favourite breakfast dish. He's been making it for us for years and it's just too good not to share with you! It's an incredibly simple dish that focuses on the individual flavours of each ingredient – so use the freshest and best tomatoes you can find. It's traditionally served over toast, but it's also an amazing sauce for pasta or rice and I'm also a huge fan of pouring it over my Quinoa and Turmeric Fritters (page 50).

Serves 4

40 cherry tomatoes (about 700g)
6 cloves of garlic
6 tablespoons olive oil
bread, to serve (I use my Superfood Bread (page 80))
salt and pepper

Chop the tomatoes into quarters, placing them into a saucepan.

Peel and crush the garlic and add that to the saucepan along with the olive oil, salt and pepper.

Cook the tomatoes for 20 minutes. For the first 5 minutes use a high heat, then allow them to simmer for the next 15, stirring the pan every few minutes until the tomatoes are nice and thick.

Spread the tomatoes over slices of bread and enjoy!

To store, allow the tomatoes to cool before placing them in an airtight container in the fridge. They'll last a few days like this.

CUCUMBER AND AVOCADO ROLLS

These cucumber and avocado rolls make the best appetizers or snacks. They're unbelievably simple to put together and only really require three ingredients – cucumbers, avocados and limes – all of which are easy to find anywhere. They're also a great picnic food in the summer as they're very refreshing thanks to the juicy lime and cool strips of cucumber.

makes about 30 rolls

2 cucumbers

2 avocados

juice of 2 limes

2 tablespoons olive oil

salt and pepper

Use a potato peeler to peel the green skin off the cucumber and discard. Peel thick pieces of cucumber, starting from one side and then from the other. You want to avoid the very middle of the cucumber as it's too flimsy to hold the rolls.

Once both cucumbers have been peeled, roll each slice into a tight circle (the tighter they are, the better they stay together).

Slice the avocados into small cubes and fill each roll with avocado (again, the fuller and more compact it is, the better it holds together).

Once all the rolls have been made, drizzle the lime juice and olive oil over the top of them and sprinkle on the salt and pepper.

Top tip

You can also try adding some of my Classic Hummus (page 102) instead of avocados in some of the rolls, if you want two different options.

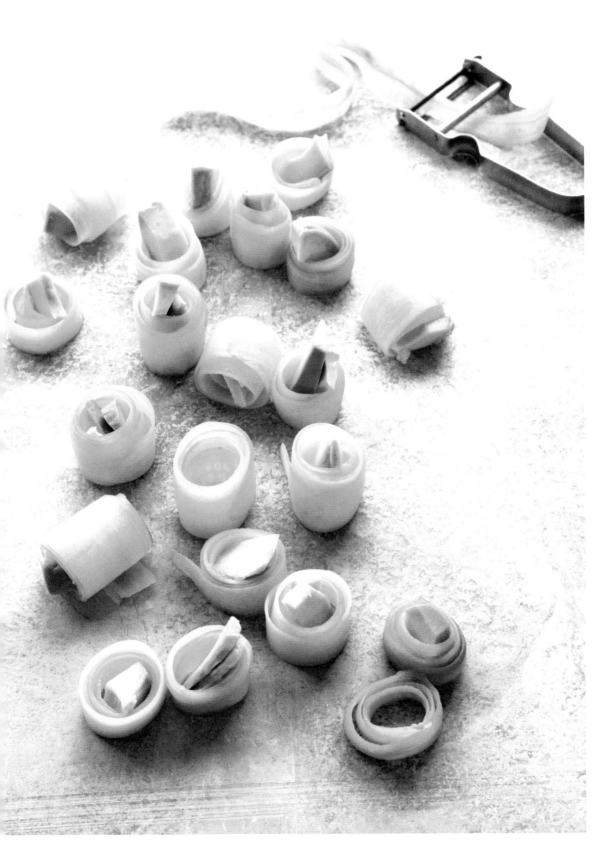

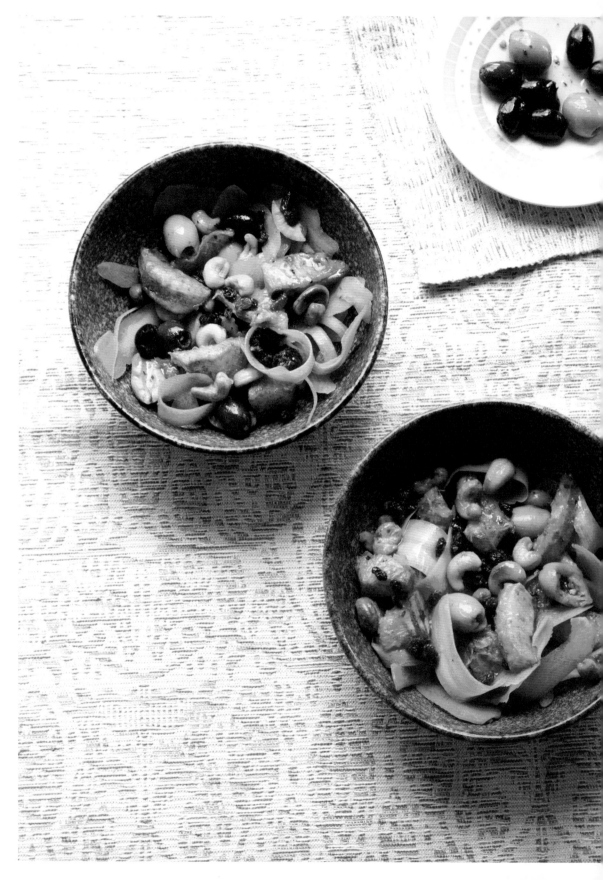

CARROT, ORANGE AND CASHEW SALAD

I'm not normally a fan of fruit in salads, but it really works here as the orange pieces are sautéed with date syrup and cumin, which totally changes their texture and taste. They lose their acidity and become soft enough to blend perfectly with the other ingredients. The salad is then dressed with orange juice too and it all has a wonderfully sweet feel to it.

Serves 4

4 carrots
1 mug raisins (200g)
5 oranges
1 teaspoon ground cumin
2 teaspoons date or maple syrup
1 mug cashews (200g)
1 mug pitted olives (180g)
salt and pepper

Peel the outside of the carrots and discard that peel. Then peel the rest of the carrots into thin slivers and place these in a large bowl.

Next, put the raisins into a bowl of boiling water and let them soak while everything else is prepared. This makes them much plumper and juicier.

Peel four of the oranges, taking the pith off as well.

Chop the inside of the oranges into bite-sized segments and place these into a saucepan with the cumin and date syrup – they don't need any oil as they have their own juice.

Sauté the oranges on a medium heat for about 5 minutes, until they're really nice and soft. Then pour them, and all the juices in the pan, over the carrots.

Now place the cashews into the same pan, so that they can soak up the orange flavour, and cook them on a medium heat for about 3 minutes until they go slightly brown, then add these to the salad too.

Squeeze the juice of the fifth orange onto the salad and mix in the olives. Drain the raisins and stir them in too with some salt and pepper before serving.

Top tip

As you peel the carrots, twist each one as you go so that the strips stay thin. If you only peel from one place, then the strips will be very wide.

BEETROOT CARPACCIO

This Beetroot Carpaccio is one of the most beautiful dishes in the book! The vibrant pink strips of beetroot just look so incredible against the green leaves of rocket, while the dressing makes the whole thing shine. It's my go-to starter dish when I'm hosting a dinner as it looks so incredible, and of course it tastes amazing too; plus it's just as easy to make this for eight or twelve people as it is for four people.

Serves 4

2 large beetroots
2 tablespoons maple syrup
2 tablespoons olive oil
1 tablespoon apple cider vinegar
handful of rocket
salt

Start by roasting the beetroots whole, with their skins on, in a 210°C (fan 190°C) oven. They will take about 45 minutes to cook. You don't need to add any olive oil.

After this time, take them out of the oven and leave them on one side to cool.

Once cool, peel the skin off and then use a potato peeler to thinly slice the beetroot into carpaccio strips.

Lay the strips across a plate.

Next, mix together the maple syrup, olive oil and apple cider vinegar in a mug before drizzling it across the carpaccio.

It's nice to let it marinate and soften for about 10 minutes before serving, so that the flavours soak in and the beetroot strips soften a little more.

Finally, sprinkle some salt over the top and then add a handful of rocket with a little more olive oil.

Top tip

If it's cold, try laying the carpaccio strips over a bed of hot, sautéed spinach instead of rocket for a more warming meal.

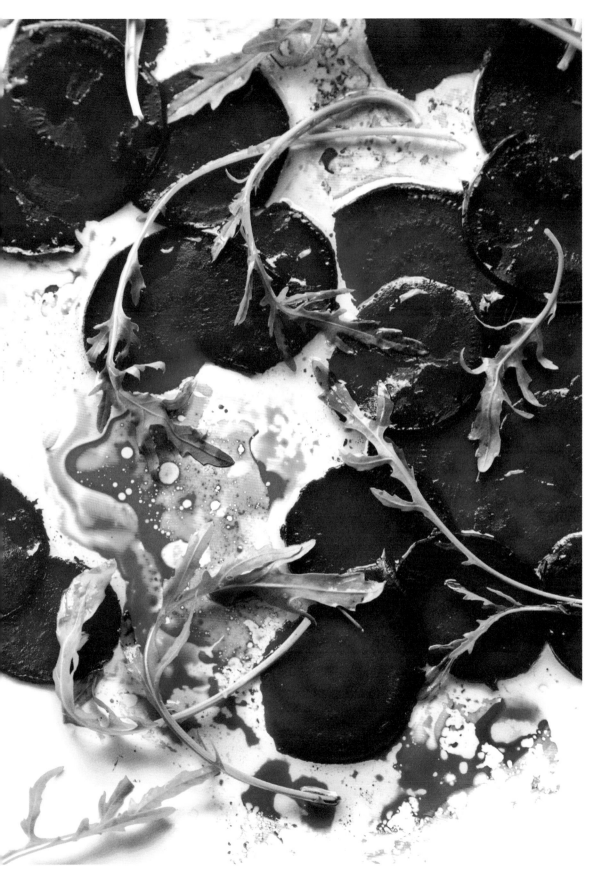

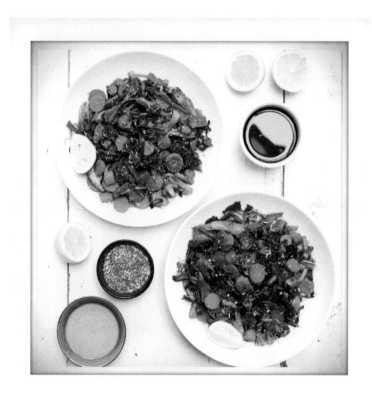

easiest weekday supper

CLASSIC STIR-FRY

This stir-fry is one of my favourite quick dinners as it's so easy to make, yet it's incredibly rich in flavours and textures. My favourite thing about it is the rich dressing made of tahini, tamari and lemon – it coats all the veggies in goodness and makes them sing with flavour! Each serving of this gives you five awesome portions of veggies too, so you'll be doing amazing things for your body while enjoying every bite.

Serves 4

4 carrots
16 long-stemmed broccoli
coconut oil
2–3cm slice of purple cabbage
two dozen chestnut mushrooms
2 red peppers
4 servings of noodles (about 300g) (I like buckwheat)
1 bag of spinach (about 250g)
3 tablespoons tamari
3 tablespoons tahini
juice of 3 lemons
3 tablespoons dried mixed herbs
salt

Start by peeling the carrots, then slice them into thin round pieces. Next, chop the broccoli stems into roughly three long segments.

Place the carrot slices and broccoli into a large wok or frying pan with 2 tablespoons coconut oil and allow them to start cooking on a medium to high heat.

Once they are cooking, slice the cabbage into thin threads, the mushrooms into rough quarters and the red pepper into small cubes. Then place them into the frying pan to cook with the carrot and broccoli.

Now, put the noodles on to cook.

Once the noodles are nearly cooked, stir the spinach into the stir-fry along with the tamari, tahini, lemon juice, herbs and salt. Drain the noodles and finally stir them into the veggies before serving and enjoying!

Top tip

If you don't have any noodles, try using my Classic Mashed Potato recipe (page 130) in their place – it's so delicious. All the veggies in this can be substituted for something else too, depending on what you have available.

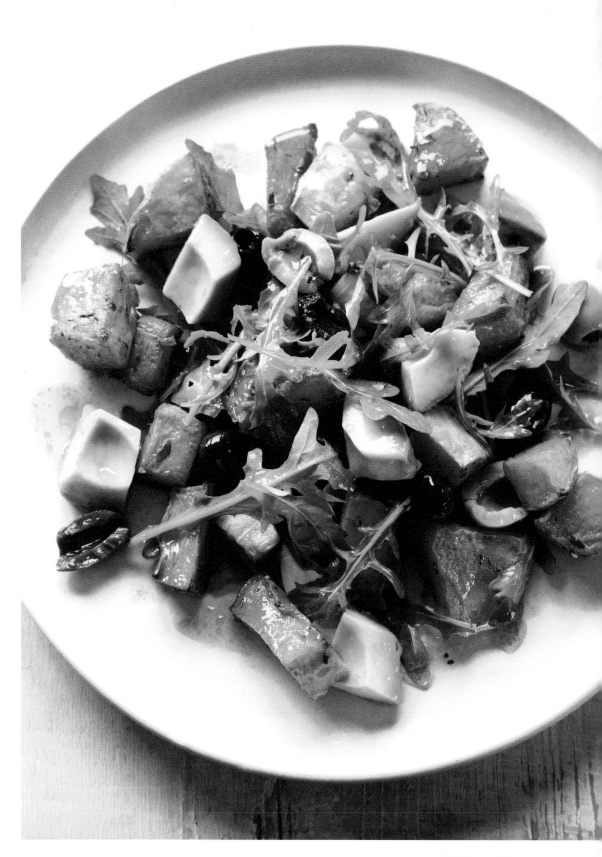

ROASTED SQUASH, OLIVE, AVOCADO AND ROCKET SALAD

This is a wonderfully simple salad, but it's full of flavours from the paprika-infused squash cubes, the salty olives, creamy avocado and peppery rocket. It's then all dressed with a tamari and apple cider vinegar dressing, which really brings it to life.

Serves 4

I large butternut squash (about 1kg)
olive oil
I tablespoon paprika
I tablespoon dried mixed herbs, such as herbes de Provence
2 bags of rocket (about 150g)
I mug pitted olives (180g)
2 avocados

For the dressing

I tablespoon tamari
2 tablespoons apple cider vinegar
2 tablespoons olive oil
salt and pepper

Preheat the oven to 200°C (fan 180°C).

Peel the butternut squash, then slice it into small bite-sized pieces.

Place the pieces into a baking tray and drizzle them with olive oil, salt and pepper, plus the paprika and dried herbs, mixing everything well to ensure it's all seasoned.

Bake the squash for about 40 minutes. Once it's nice and soft, leave it to one side to cool.

For the dressing

Make the dressing by mixing all the ingredients together with a little salt and pepper, to taste.

Mix the rocket with the dressing and olives, before cutting the avocados into small cubes and adding them to the salad with the squash once it's cool.

Top tip

You can make this as a warm salad in the winter by replacing the rocket with steamed spinach.

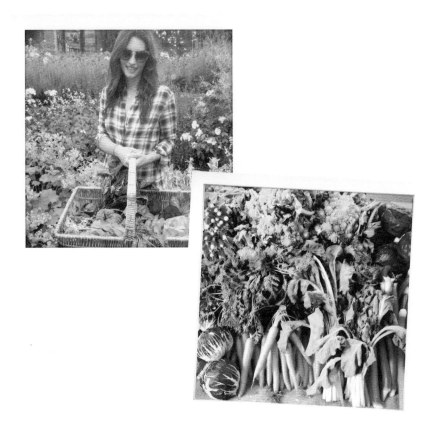

'You have helped me heal myself
and make peace with food and with
my body.' – Sophie

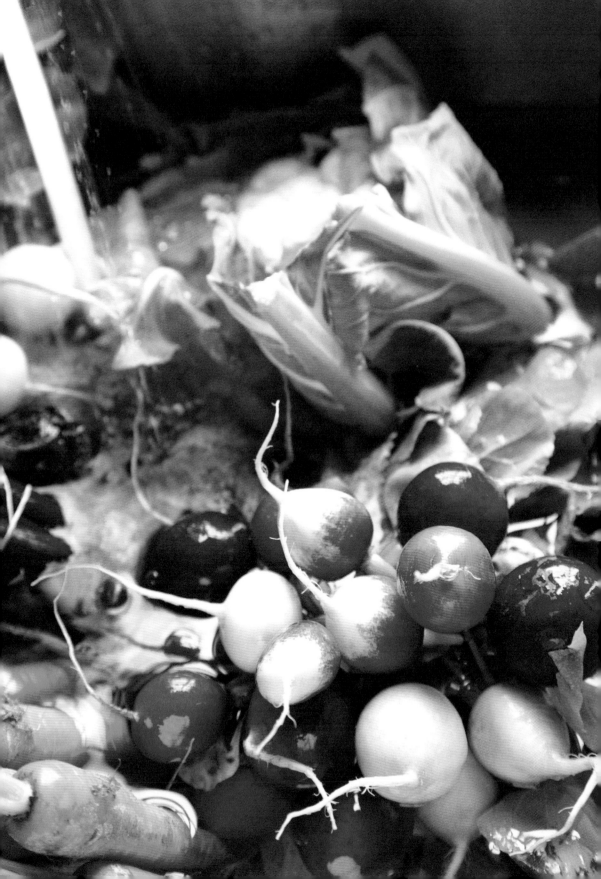

BROCCOLI AND AVOCADO SALAD

This salad is a favourite recipe from the blog and it's one of my first ever recipes too. The beauty of it really lies in its perfect simplicity; it's such an uncomplicated dish, so all the individual flavours and textures really shine through. I love how the avocado melts against the ever-so-slightly crunchy broccoli and fresh coriander leaves, while the tahini, lime and tamari dressing add a wonderful tangy touch. This is healthy eating at its best: simple, delicious, quick and inexpensive. I love this served with homemade Hummus (page 102) and some Sweet Potato Wedges (page 132).

Serves 4

For the salad
1½ heads of broccoli
3 ripe avocados
handful of fresh coriander

For the dressing
juice of 3 limes (about 30ml juice)
2 tablespoons tahini
2 teaspoons tamari
3 tablespoons olive oil
2 teaspoons honey or maple syrup
sprinkling of salt

For the salad

Start by slicing the broccoli into small, bite-sized pieces. Then steam these in a steamer for about 7 minutes, until cooked but a little crunchy. If you don't have a steamer, you can boil the broccoli. Place to one side to cool.

Slice the avocados in half, peel their skin away and remove their stones. Then slice the flesh into small cubes.

Chop the coriander into tiny pieces and mix with the avocado and broccoli in a salad bowl.

For the dressing

Squeeze the limes into a mug and add the tahini, tamari, olive oil, honey and salt. Stir the dressing well and the drizzle it over the salad.

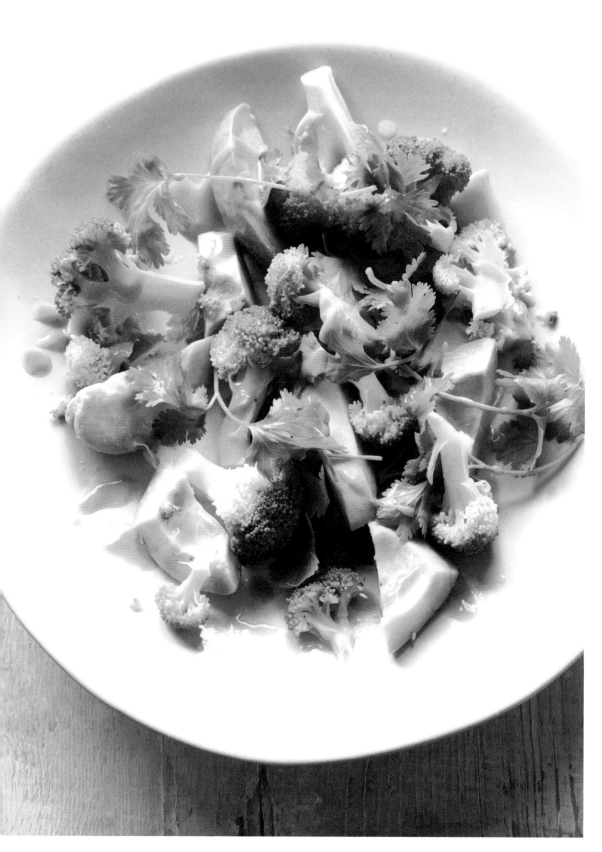

STUFFED CHESTNUT MUSHROOMS

I've tried stuffed Portobello mushrooms so many times, but they always throw up the same issue – way too much water! Every time you bake them, they ooze so much water that the stuffing gets filtered down and it's good, but it's not amazing. So I tried using chestnut mushrooms one day and it instantly solved all my problems, they hold together perfectly so they look beautiful and taste so much better. My favourite thing about this dish though is the way that the sun-dried tomato and pine nut stuffing melts into the mushrooms as they bake, it's divine. I love serving them with my Carrot, Orange and Cashew Salad (page 139) or a side of potatoes, either a bowl of Classic Mashed Potato (page 130) or lots of Sweet Potato Wedges (page 132).

Serves 4

12 chestnut mushrooms
1 mug sun-dried tomatoes (180g)
big handful of fresh basil
¾ mug pine nuts (100g)
2 tablespoons tahini
juice of 1 lime
salt and pepper

Preheat the oven to 200°C (fan 180°C).

Remove the stalks of the mushrooms and place the mushrooms on a baking tray.

Cut up the sun-dried tomatoes and basil, then mix them with the pine nuts, tahini, lime juice, salt and pepper.

Stuff the mix into the mushrooms, sprinkling any leftover mix around the mushrooms on the tray to bake.

Place the mushrooms in the oven and bake for 15–20 minutes, until the mushrooms are soft and delicious.

Top tip

Try using the sun-dried tomato mix as a pasta sauce instead of in the mushrooms – it's so delicious!

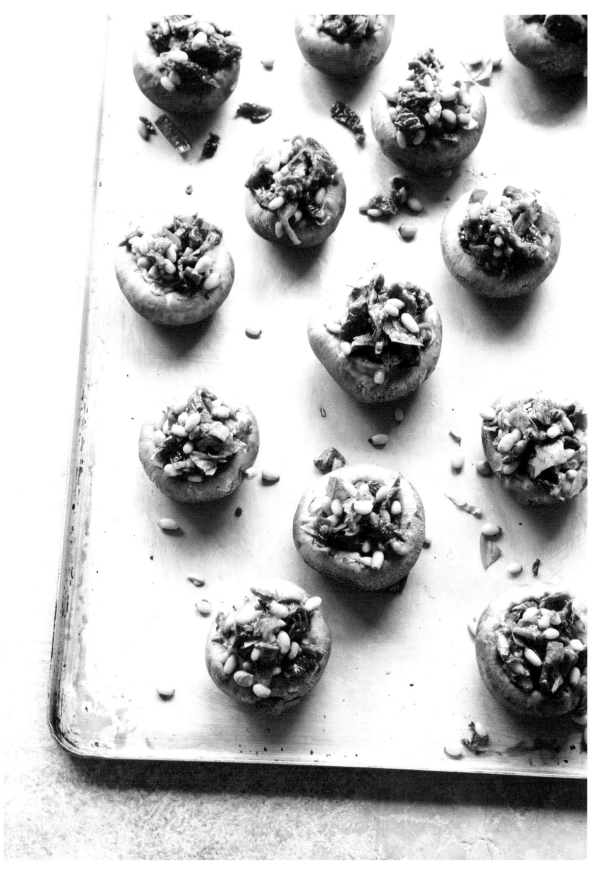

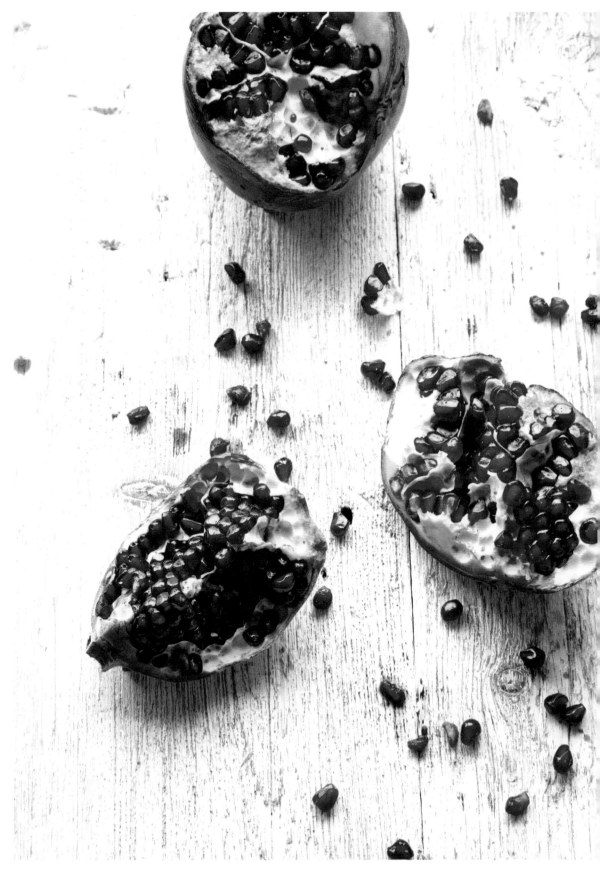

MARINATED KALE SALAD

This kale salad has a very similar dressing to the Broccoli and Avocado Salad (page 148) and it's another favourite both of mine, and of the blog. I know raw kale doesn't sound that appetising, but this is another recipe where you just have to trust me and try it! The dressing really does amazing things to the kale leaves and I'm yet to find a single person that doesn't fall in love with kale after they try this! It's a great side dish for almost anything. I especially love it with my Easy Roast Veggies (page 128).

Serves 4

big bag of kale (250g)
2 limes
4 tablespoons tahini
3 tablespoons tamari
2 tablespoons olive oil
½ mug pomegranate seeds (120g)
salt and pepper

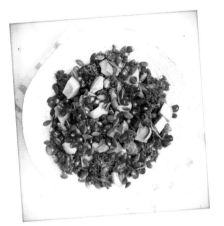

Tear the kale leaves off their stems into a salad bowl.

Juice the limes, then add the juice to the bowl along with the tahini, tamari and olive oil.

Use your hands to firmly massage the kale with the dressing, really working it into each leaf. After a couple of minutes you should feel the kale wilt and soften.

At this point, add the pomegranate seeds.

Top tip

Try bulking out this salad by adding some roasted veggies, like sweet potatoes, aubergines or carrots. You can also add avocado for an instant hit of creamy deliciousness, or some pumpkin or sunflower seeds for a protein-rich crunch.

WARM WINTER SALAD

This salad was one of the first recipes I created for the book and I've been coming back to it time and time again ever since. I just love the mix of flavours and textures here, from the wilted spinach and roasted aubergine to the crunchy pine nuts, sweet sun-dried tomatoes and creamy tahini sauce. It's a pretty filling dish, but if you're feeling really hungry, then try serving it with some brown rice or quinoa with a little lemon drizzled over. It's one of my favourite meals to make for friends when I'm after an easy kitchen supper and it's always such a winner.

Serves 4

4 small aubergines (600g)
olive oil
1 tablespoon dried mixed herbs (I love herbes de Provence)
2 bags of spinach (about 500g)
4 tablespoons tahini
juice of 1 lime
2 mugs sun-dried tomatoes (360g)
1 mug pine nuts (100g)
salt and pepper

Preheat the oven to 200°C (fan 180°C).

Slice the aubergines into thin strips about 7.5mm thick.

Place the strips on a baking tray with a generous amount of olive oil, the dried herbs, salt and pepper.

Bake for 20 minutes.

About 5 minutes before the aubergines finish, place the spinach into a large frying pan with a little olive oil, salt and pepper and allow it to wilt. Once it's wilted, add the tahini, lime juice and sun-dried tomatoes.

In a separate pan, toast the pine nuts for a minute or two, being sure not to let them burn – they don't need any oil to cook as they contain enough of their own oil.

Add the aubergine and pine nuts to the spinach pan and mix well before serving.

Top tip

Watch out for the ingredients of sun-dried tomatoes – they can often contain lots of sugars and preservatives. If you can only find these ones, then rinse them in boiling water before using them.

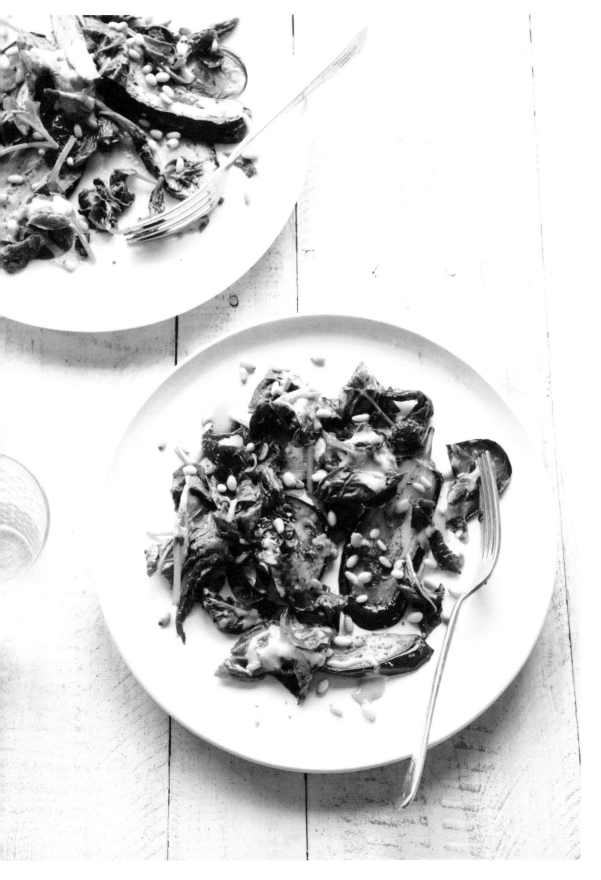

VEGGIE LASAGNE

Growing up, lasagne was my favourite meal. I just couldn't get enough of it and it's one of the foods that I missed the most when I changed my diet, so I was unbelievably excited when I created this recipe for Veggie Lasagne. The most exciting bit about this recipe is the cheese layer, which is made out of butternut squash and coconut milk. It might not sound that exciting, but it tastes absolutely heavenly! It freezes beautifully, so make double and freeze half.

Serves 4

2 large butternut squash (2kg)
3 cloves of garlic, peeled and crushed
4 dozen cherry tomatoes, halved
4 red peppers, cut into small bite-sized pieces
olive oil
500g mushrooms, thinly sliced
8 lasagne sheets (I use brown rice lasagne)
½ x 400ml tin coconut milk
salt and pepper

Peel the squash and cut them into small pieces, then steam these for 20 minutes until they're really soft and tender.

Sauté the garlic in a saucepan with the tomatoes, peppers and some olive oil on a low heat.

Add the mushrooms to the pan to cook for about 10 minutes. At this point, take the pan off the heat and leave it to one side.

While everything is cooking, precook the lasagne sheets by placing them in a pan of boiling water, with a little olive oil to stop them sticking together, for 10 minutes (check the back of your pasta packet for details though, as these can vary and some don't need precooking).

Once the squash has finished steaming, add it to a food processor with the coconut milk and some salt and pepper. Blend until smooth and creamy.

Preheat the oven to 200°C (fan 180°C).

Finally, assemble the lasagne! Place a layer of mushrooms and tomatoes on the bottom of a baking dish, then add a layer of the squash purée, a layer of pasta, a second layer of mushrooms and tomatoes, a second layer of pasta and finally a second layer of squash purée. Cover the top of the baking dish in tin foil and bake for about 20 minutes until golden brown.

CAULIFLOWER AND POTATO CURRY

This curry has so much flavour – it's pretty incredible. You can really taste the wide ra⁓
of spices in each bite, which I love, from the turmeric to the cumin, mustard seeds, ginger,
garlic and jalapeño. Together, all these spices make the potatoes and cauliflower taste
unbelievable. This is a really simple dish to make too and it's a great meal to serve to lots of
people as there's minimal chopping involved in it!

Serves 4

about 24 Charlotte potatoes (1.4kg)
1 head of cauliflower
3 x 400g tins of tomatoes
1 x 400ml tin of coconut milk
3 cloves of garlic, peeled and crushed
3 tablespoons mustard seeds
3 tablespoons ground turmeric
3 tablespoons ground cumin
3 tablespoons ground ginger
2 jalapeño peppers
olive oil
1 bag of spinach (about 250g)
brown rice, to serve
salt and pepper

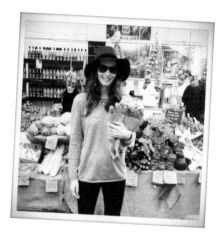

Start by boiling the potatoes for 15 minutes, until they are softening. After
15 minutes, drain the potatoes and leave them to one side to cool.

Once the potatoes are cool, chop them into quarters or sixths, depending
on their size; they want to be big bite-sized chunks.

Slice the cauliflower into chunks and place it all in a deep saucepan with
the potatoes, tinned tomatoes and coconut milk and begin to heat gently.

Next, put the garlic into a frying pan along with the mustard seeds,
turmeric, cumin, ginger, salt and pepper. Then chop the jalapeño peppers
into tiny pieces, discarding their seeds and placing the pieces into the
frying pan. Cover everything in a generous amount of olive oil and cook on
a high heat for a couple of minutes until the mustard seeds begin to pop.
At this point, pour everything into the potato and cauliflower pan.

Put the lid on the pan and allow it to simmer for 45 minutes to an hour,
until the potatoes are nice and soft. At this point, stir in the spinach and
allow it to wilt before serving on a bed of brown rice.

'You have helped me on my quest to changing my mindset, realising that nourishment and treating your body well with nature's goods, changes your entire life. I honestly can't thank you enough.' – Hannah

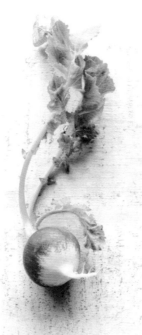

BROCCOLI WITH A TAHINI DRESSING

This is one of my favourite side dishes as it's so easy to make and goes with just about everything. The broccoli is lightly steamed, then it's covered in a creamy tahini dressing and topped with toasted cashews, so that each bite is bursting with texture and flavour.

Serves 4 as a side

500g broccoli

2 tablespoons tahini

2 tablespoons olive oil, plus extra for the cashews

2 teaspoons honey

1 mug cashew nuts (200g)

Steam the broccoli for about 7 minutes, so that it's nicely cooked but still a little crunchy.

While it steams, stir the tahini, olive oil and honey together in a mug until smooth and creamy.

Crush the cashews by pulsing them in a food processor for short 3–5 second blasts. Once they are crushed, place them in a frying pan with a little olive oil and cook for a couple of minutes until they are crunchy.

Place the cooked broccoli on a serving plate, drizzle it with the tahini dressing and finally sprinkle the cashews on the top.

CLASSIC GUACAMOLE

Guacamole, like hummus, is the easiest dip to make yourself, so you really don't need to buy the processed versions in supermarkets. It's a really easy thing to serve friends as a snack, either with crudités, flax crisps or rice cakes, and I also pair it with my Marinated Kale Salad (page 153) or Warm Winter Salad (page 154).

Makes 1 large bowl

4 ripe avocados (450g)

half a dozen tomatoes (140g)

1 large jalapeño pepper

handful of fresh coriander, finely chopped

optional: I don't love garlic and onions in my guacamole, but if you do, then please add these in

juice of 3 limes (about 30ml)

salt and pepper

First cut the avocados in half and scoop out their flesh, placing it into a bowl. Use a fork to mash them.

Chop the tomatoes and the jalapeño pepper into tiny pieces (discard the seeds of the pepper). Stir everything into the mashed avocado with the lime juice, salt and pepper.

COURGETTE NOODLES WITH AVOCADO PESTO

This is one of my favourite speedy weekday suppers, and yes, this is what I'm eating on the cover! It only takes 10 minutes and requires almost no chopping, which I love! Courgette noodles are the best pasta replacement as they have the exact same texture, but they're a little lighter and packed full of vitamins. They taste incredible tossed in this minty avocado and brazil nut sauce with a heap of sautéed mushrooms on the top.

Serves 4

For the noodles
4 courgettes
two dozen chestnut mushrooms
olive oil

For the avocado pesto
1 mug brazil nuts (120g)
4 avocados
4 tablespoons olive oil
large handful of fresh mint leaves
juice of 4 limes
salt and pepper

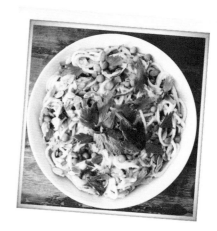

For the noodles

Start by making the courgette noodles by simply putting the courgettes through your spiralizer. Place the noodles to one side and begin the mushrooms.

Cut the mushrooms into thin slices, drizzle them with olive oil, and then gently heat them in a large frying pan for about 5 minutes, until they're nice and soft.

For the avocado pesto

While the mushrooms cook, place the brazil nuts in a food processor and blend for a minute or two, until they're totally crushed. Then add in the avocado flesh, olive oil, mint leaves, juiced lime and a sprinkling of salt and pepper and blend again.

Either mix the noodles and sauce together in a bowl raw and then add the mushrooms, or add the sauce and noodles to the mushrooms in the frying pan and gently heat for a couple of minutes to warm the dish up and soften the noodles a little.

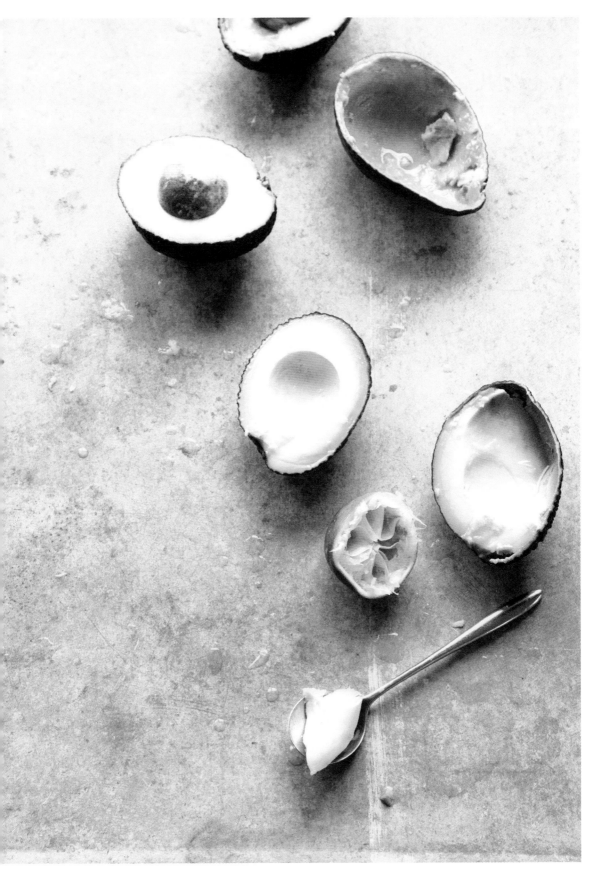

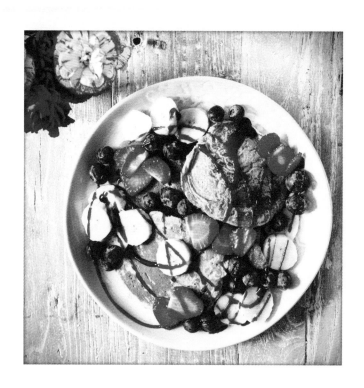

my favourite breakfast

SWEET POTATO PANCAKES

These Sweet Potato Pancakes are pretty amazing; they only contain five ingredients – all of which are great for you. Sweet potato is the best ingredient too as it holds the pancakes together, while also adding a great flavour. I love serving these with my Strawberry Jam (page 187), a little Apple Purée (page 19) and some fresh fruit.

makes 12 pancakes
1 small sweet potato (200g)
⅔ mug oat milk (200ml)
1 mug brown rice flour (200g)
2 tablespoons honey
1 teaspoon ground cinnamon
coconut oil, for greasing

Peel the sweet potato, discard the skin and chop the rest of the potato into small pieces.

Either steam or boil the sweet potato chunks for about 10 minutes, until they're really soft.

Then place them into a blender with the oat milk, flour, honey and cinnamon and blend for 30 seconds or so until the mix is totally smooth.

Place a non-stick frying pan on the stove and grease it with coconut oil, then allow it to get really hot before placing about 2 tablespoons worth of batter in it.

Use a spoon to shape the batter into a circle and then allow it to cook for 2–3 minutes, until the top of it no longer looks like runny batter and is starting to firm. Flip the pancake over and allow it to cook on the other side.

Continue until you've used up all the batter.

Top tip
Make sure that you cook the first side for long enough. It's tough to be patient, but if you're not then they won't flip properly.

BEETROOT CHOCOLATE CAKE *with Coconut Frosting*

This cake is so awesome. I made it for a while at my cooking classes and everyone always loved it. Again, I know it's strange to put veggies into a dessert, but here it creates something very special as the sponge has a slightly earthy taste that contrasts so perfectly with the coconut icing. Each bite is wonderfully rich and decadent, yet full of goodness. I love this served with some of my Banana Ice Cream (page 198).

Makes 1 cake (12 slices)

For the cake

1 large beetroot (250g)
2 mugs buckwheat flour (400g)
1 mug apple purée (360g)
  (recipe on page 19)
1 mug maple syrup (300ml)
6 tablespoons raw cacao powder
pinch of salt
coconut oil, for greasing

For the frosting

100g coconut cream
1 tablespoon almond butter
(recipe on page 24)
2 tablespoons maple syrup
1 tablespoon raw cacao powder

For the cake

Using a steamer, steam the beetroot whole (with its skins on) for about an hour, until it's very soft. If you don't have a steamer, you can boil the beetroot. Then take it out of the steamer and allow it to cool.

Once the beetroot is cool, peel its skin off and chop off the head.

Preheat the oven to 190°C (fan 170°C).

Cut up the flesh of the beetroot, place it into a food processor and blend until a smooth purée forms.

Add the purée to a mixing bowl with all the other ingredients and mix well until perfectly smooth and creamy.

Grease a 20–25cm cake tin with coconut oil, then pour in the mix and bake for about 20 minutes until you can pull a knife out of the centre totally clean.

For the frosting

As the cake cools, make the icing. Simply place the coconut cream in a bowl or mug with 3 tablespoons boiling water and stir until it's totally melted. Add this to a blender with the almond butter, maple syrup and cacao and blend until smooth.

Pour the icing over the cake and serve!

Top tip

Try making this cake as brownies, they're amazing!

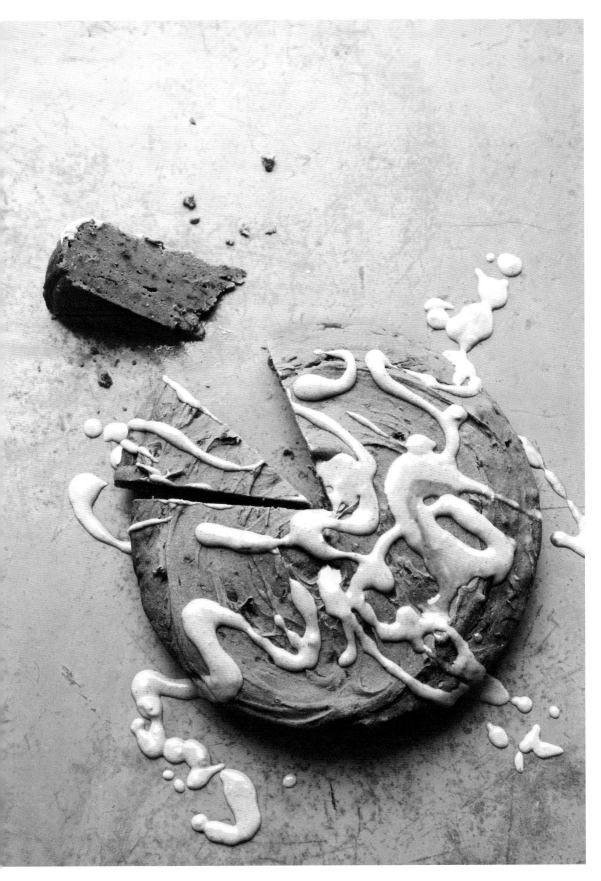

SWEET POTATO BROWNIES

These brownies have consistently been the most popular recipe on my blog. They've had more than double the amount of hits than the next most popular recipe and I've seen thousands of my readers' photographs of them on Instagram! There's a good reason for all this love, though – the brownies are divine. I know it sounds strange to put vegetables into sweet dishes, but sweet potatoes taste more like dessert anyway and they create the gooiest consistency!

Makes 10–12 brownies

2 medium-large sweet potatoes (600g)

14 Medjool dates, pitted

⅔ mug ground almonds (80g)

½ mug buckwheat or brown rice flour (100g)

4 tablespoons raw cacao powder

3 tablespoons maple syrup

pinch of salt

Preheat the oven to 180°C (fan 160°C).

Peel the sweet potatoes. Cut them into chunks and place into a steamer for about 20 minutes, until they become really soft.

Once they are perfectly soft and beginning to fall apart, remove them and add them to a food processor with the pitted dates. Blend until a smooth, creamy mix forms.

Put the remaining ingredients into a bowl, before mixing in the sweet potato and date combination. Stir well.

Place the mix into a lined baking dish and cook for about 20–30 minutes, until you can pierce the brownie cake with a fork and bring it out dry. Remove the tray and allow it to cool for about 10 minutes. This is really important, as the brownies need this time to stick together!

Top tip

If you don't have any raw cacao powder, then you can use conventional cocoa powder, but you'll need to at least double the quantity.

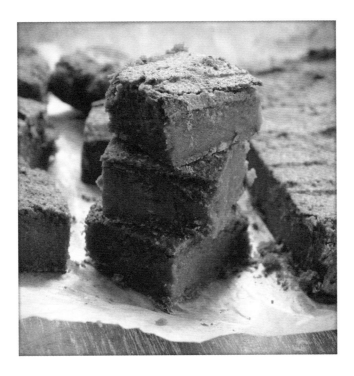

gooey bites of heaven

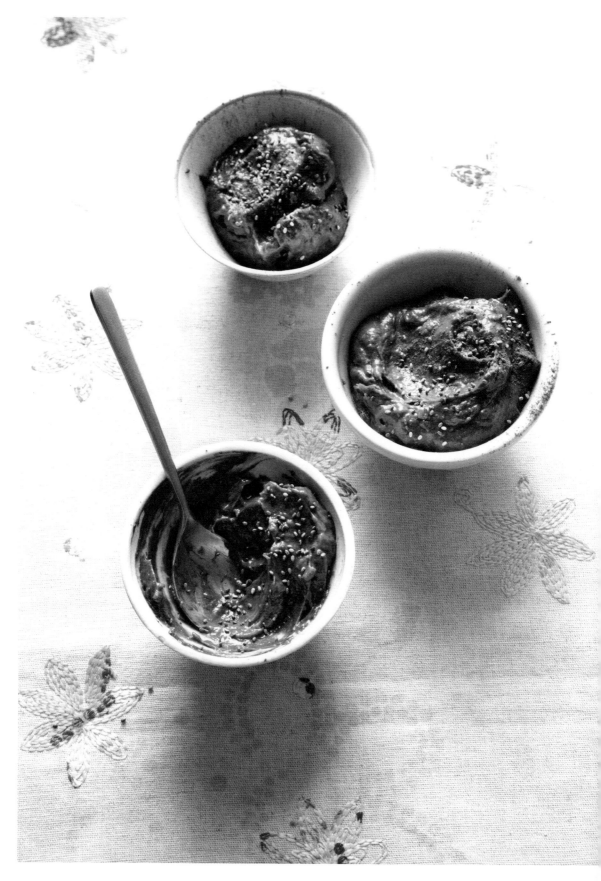

EASY AVOCADO CHOCOLATE MOUSSE

These little chocolate mousses are one of the best speedy snacks or desserts. There's no cooking or chopping involved either, so they go from fridge to plate in less than 5 minutes! The secret ingredient here is avocado, which gives them the thick, decadently creamy feel. The avocado flavour totally disappears though under the rich chocolate flavours of the cacao, the nutty almond butter, the sweet banana and the caramel-like dates, so I promise you won't know that you're eating vegetables in your pudding!

Serves 4

2 ripe avocados
4 really ripe bananas, peeled (400g)
12 Medjool dates, pitted
4 tablespoons almond butter (recipe on page 24)
5 heaped teaspoons raw cacao powder
optional: drizzle of maple syrup
optional: sprinkle of chia seeds

Slice the avocados in half, peel their skin away and remove their stones. Then place the flesh into a food processor.

Add all the remaining ingredients to the food processor with a splash of water and the maple syrup, if using, then blend into a smooth, delicious mixture. Divide the mixture among four ramekins or little glasses and sprinkle over the chia seeds, if using.

Keep chilled in the fridge until you're ready to eat.

CLASSIC CARROT CAKE *with Caramel Frosting*

This double-layered carrot cake with a creamy caramel-like icing is pretty special. One of the really nice things about it is that the sponge is very light so you feel incredibly energised after enjoying it, which I love – although it does mean that you'll be tempted to eat four or five slices in a row!

makes 1 cake (12 slices)

For the cake

2 mugs brown rice or buckwheat
    flour (400g)
1 mug ground almonds (120g)
2 tablespoons chia seeds
⅓ mug raisins (65g)
2 slices of pineapple (225g)
1 mug almond milk (300ml)
    (recipe on page 20)
½ mug maple syrup (150ml)
3 carrots (250g)
coconut oil, for greasing

For the frosting

3 large bananas, peeled (350g)
10 Medjool dates, pitted
2 tablespoons almond butter
    (recipe on page 24)
1 tablespoon coconut oil
1 teaspoon ground cinnamon

For the cake

Preheat the oven to 180°C (fan 160°C).

Pour the brown rice/buckwheat flour into a mixing bowl with the ground almonds, chia seeds and raisins.

Place the pineapple, almond milk and maple syrup into a blender and blend until smooth. Once it's totally smooth, pour the mix into the mixing bowl with the dry ingredients.

Next, peel and grate the carrots using the fine side of a box grater. Stir the carrot into the mixing bowl and ensure that it's all thoroughly mixed so that it forms a smooth batter.

Grease two x 24cm cake tins with coconut oil and evenly pour the mixture into both.

Bake for about 30 minutes, until the tops turn a golden brown.

Once the cakes are cooked, remove them from the oven and leave them to cool for about 10 minutes on a cooling rack (this is really important as the cake finishes setting at this point).

For the frosting

As the cake cools, make the icing. Place everything into a blender with 4 tablespoons water and blend until a smooth, creamy mix forms.

Once the cakes have cooled, divide the icing between the two cakes and then ice the tops.

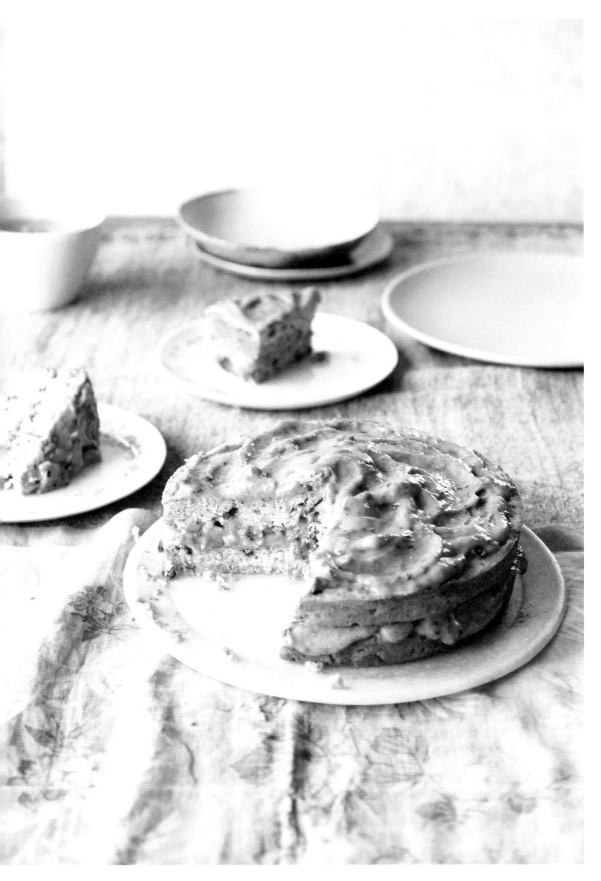

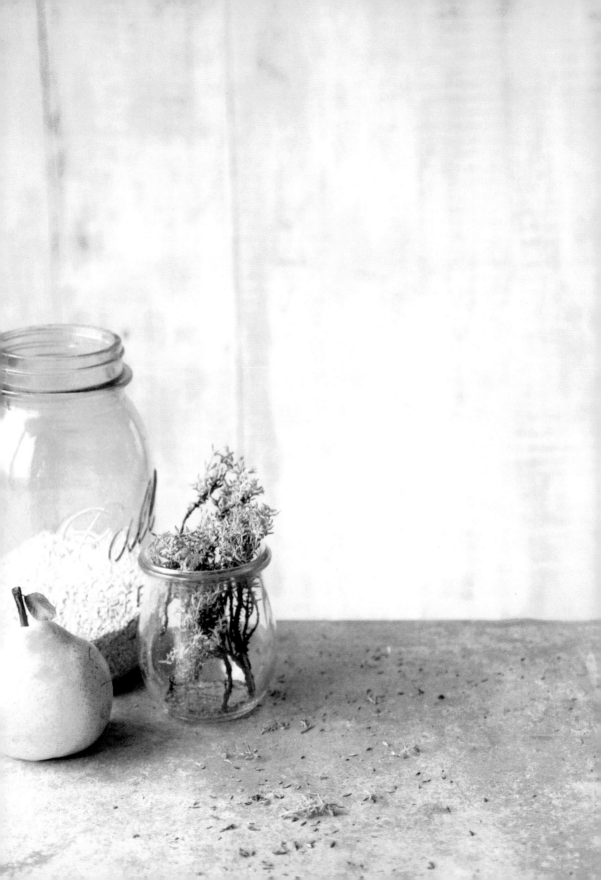

FRUIT

nature's candy

BAKED APPLES WITH COCONUT CREAM

WAFFLES

SIMPLE MANGO AND CASHEW MOUSSE

BLUEBERRY MUFFINS

STRAWBERRY JAM

DATE PURÉE

APPLE AND BLACKBERRY CRUMBLE

BAKED BANANAS STUFFED WITH MELTED DARK CHOCOLATE

BERRY CHEESECAKE

BANOFFEE PIE

KEY LIME PIE

BANANA, BERRY AND CARAMEL ICE CREAM

ICE LOLLIES

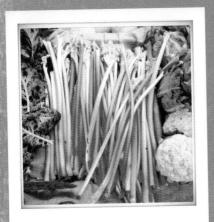

'You taught me how to live a plant-based and healthy lifestyle and most of all that eating healthy can be fun! I honestly cannot express my gratitude at how you have helped change my life. Thank you for helping me realise my potential and for inspiring me!' – Connie

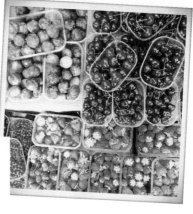

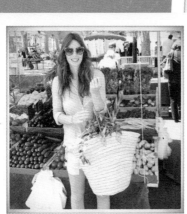

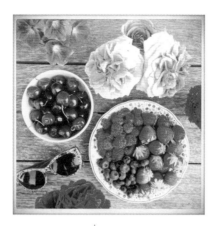

fruit

Fruit really is nature's candy – so wonderfully bright, vibrant and sweet. I really don't think there is anything more beautiful than a bowl of rainbow-coloured fruit; seriously, it really looks just like Skittles! As you know, however, I didn't used to like fruit. It was primarily a texture thing for me, so I taught myself to love it by using fruit in inventive ways so that I didn't realise it was there!

I realise this might sound very strange, but doing this achieved two awesome things. Firstly, and most importantly, it taught me that fruit is actually delicious. Secondly, and most excitingly, it showed me that fruit was actually incredibly versatile and could be used in lots of ways that I'd never thought of before – mainly to make seemingly very unhealthy things into incredible healthy ones! I mean, who knew that if you froze sliced bananas and then blended them, that they would make ice cream, or that you could use mashed bananas, dates or apple purée instead of eggs in baking? I was also excited to discover that I could blend fruit into the most delicious desserts, so that I could eat fruit without realising it – it's just so simple. So if you're not a big fan of fruit, I'd recommend blending it as a way to start enjoying it and getting more fruit into your diet. For instance, you can do simple thing like mixing mangoes with cashews to make the silkiest, richest, most decadent mousse ever (page 184)!

Fruit now lies at the heart of so many of my favourite dishes, from puddings to baking, granola to smoothies. It's just such a versatile ingredient and once you get creative, you can come up with so many wonderful and unexpected things. I use apple purée to add a little sweetness to savoury dishes, from Hash Browns (page 130) to Falafels (page 107), while I use date syrup to add sweetness to my Baked Beans (page 112). I add oranges to salads, like my Carrot, Orange and Cashew Salad (page 139), and I add mango to my dipping sauce for my Spring Rolls (page 53). Honestly, I never would have believed you four years ago if you told me that I'd be adding fruit to everything, but I just love it and can't get enough of it.

Of course, fruit also takes centre stage in all my

favourite sweet dishes too. My all-time favourite
desserts are now my Baked Apples stuffed with
raisins, pecans and coconut sugar (page 180)
and Banana Ice Cream (page 192) – both of
these recipes focus primarily on fruit and it's just
amazing. It's so fun to find new ways to eat your
favourite foods, as baking the apples or puréeing
the banana totally change their normal taste
and texture, opening up a whole new world of
delicious goodness.

The most exciting discovery I had on my
fruit adventure, though, was dates. Now I know
that dates don't look especially sexy – after all
they're small, brown and squishy – but they
taste like heaven and they are incredible in
cooking. Honestly, I have to ration myself with
them sometimes as I could eat hundreds and
hundreds – they're just too delicious. To me they
taste exactly like caramel, so they're the perfect
addition to any sweet recipe. Not only do they
act as a natural sweetener, they also work to stick
all the ingredients together as they're naturally
so gooey. I can hear lots of you asking me about
the sugar content at this point! Dates do contain
sugar, it's true, but it's natural sugar, which just
isn't the same as refined white sugar as it doesn't
spike your blood sugar or cause inflammatory
responses in the body. Plus dates are very good for
your digestive system and contain lots of goodness
from fibre to iron, zinc, magnesium, calcium
and a whole host of other vitamins and minerals.
Getting an abundance of these vitamins and
minerals in your diet is crucial as they are essential
for all processes in your body, from repairing
your muscles and stopping cramp to keeping your
bones strong, to delivering oxygen to your cells
and giving you all the energy you need to look and
feel your best.

The other thing that's really important to stress
is that we're all only human – no matter how
healthy we are or try to be, it's totally normal to
crave sweet things, which is why I think it's so

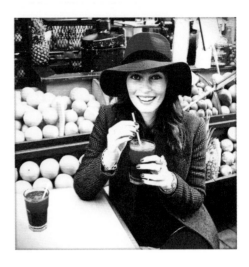

important to learn how to cook gorgeously sweet,
delicious things that look and taste amazing, but
are secretly full of goodness! When I first started
eating this way, I had no idea that you could make
desserts without refined sugar, gluten or processed
ingredients and so for three months I craved every
kind of chocolate bar and bag of sweets around,
because I felt deprived. Eating the Deliciously Ella
way just isn't about deprivation, as you know, it's
about enjoying food, and enjoying food means
enjoying sweet things. That's not to say that I
think you should eat a whole raw cheesecake every
day, it might be full of healthy ingredients, but
moderation is still a good thing. However, if you
want something sweet, don't deprive yourself or
else you'll just feel unhappy – and that's not what
we're aiming for here!

There are lots of recipes that can be made and
kept in the fridge for whenever your body asks
for something sweet. Things like the Almond and
Chia Energy Bites (page 72) and Raw Brownies
(page 89) can be left in the fridge for around
three weeks or frozen for a few months. They sate
all your cravings and leave you feeling energised

and happy, so you simply won't want to eat so much processed stuff. I try to bake something every week too, normally simple things like the Sweet Potato Brownies (page 166) or Blueberry Muffins (page 184), so that I have a great range of delicious things to snack on. However, if I don't have time to do this, then it's amazing to know that I have the energy balls or raw brownies waiting for me in the fridge.

Once I started cooking this way for my friends and family, I was amazed by how much they were enjoying my sweet treats, and how most of the time they didn't realise that they were 'healthy' treats and would finish their plateful within seconds! Take my version of Banoffee Pie (page 195), for example. It really does taste exactly like banoffee pie and you would never know that the banoffee layer is made of just dates, almond butter, banana and a little water instead of condensed milk and sugar, but trust me, you'll feel the difference in your body.

I totally understand if you don't believe me that the healthy versions of classic puddings can taste incredible. I wouldn't have believed it either before I changed the way I eat, but trust me, once you try it you'll be totally with me on this one. The Apple and Blackberry Crumble (page 189) tastes and feels identical to normal crumble, but again, you feel fantastic after eating it – less bloated, less lethargic and really healthy. It's also so good for you that you can (and I often do) eat it for breakfast!

I know sometimes the ingredients in the desserts may seem a little unconventional – I accept that it seems weird to use avocado in dessert, make ice cream with just bananas or use cashew nuts instead of cream cheese. What I would say is that if you're a sceptic, then you just have to be open-minded and forget what's in it, and trust me when I say that it's delicious. For instance, when I have friends over for dinner and they're not so sure about the way I eat and haven't tried any of my food yet, I don't tell them what's in it, but make them take a few bites, hear that they love it, and then reveal that the chocolate mousse they're eating is in fact based almost entirely on avocados. They're almost always shocked, in a good way! If you're trying to get children to eat these things, then this is a good technique as sometimes if you're weirded out by an ingredient, it clouds your judgement of the actual taste itself.

So start eating lots of fruit, as all fruits are nutritional powerhouses, packed with all the vitamins, minerals, fibre and antioxidants we need to look and feel beautiful. I hope that all the recipes you see in this chapter will encourage you to start getting creative with your fruit so that you can eat much more of it, as in our world full of processed food, nature's candy really is such a gift.

There are too many different types of fruits to give you a breakdown of all of them, but I just wanted to share a little information on my favourite fruits, which are the ones that you'll see most often in this chapter.

APPLES

Apples are one of the most versatile fruits; I use them in so many dishes. As I mentioned above, Apple Purée (page 19) is a great addition to sweet and savoury dishes as it adds sweetness while also working to stick the recipe together. I love baked apples too, they're so tender and delicious – both my Apple and Blackberry Crumble (page 189) and my Baked Apples (page 180) are regular fixtures in my weekly meals.

One of the best things about apples is that they're a great source of fibre, which helps to regulate your blood sugar levels so that you stay happy and energetic all day. All the fibre is also great for supporting your digestive system, keeping it working efficiently. Apples are high in antioxidants too, which are vital for beautiful, glowing skin. Try enjoying apple slices dipped into home-made Cacao and Hazelnut Spread (page 79), Date Purée (page 187) or Almond Butter (page 24) for an afternoon snack. They're all great options as they'll fight off that four o'clock energy slump.

BANANAS

As a child, bananas were the only fruit I'd eat. I didn't really like them, but every few weeks my mum would make me eat one, so I would play a fun game with my banana where I'd cut it into the smallest possible pieces and then play eenie meenie miney mo with them, so that it would take about an hour or so to eat it! Fortunately I've moved on from this and now gobble up a couple of bananas every day, either blending them into my smoothies, mashing them onto my Superfood Bread (page 80) with some Almond Butter (page 24) or getting creative with them to make Baked Bananas Stuffed with Melted Dark Chocolate (page 190).

Like apples, bananas are great binding agents, so they also work as fantastic egg replacements, which is how I've used them in recipes like my Waffles (page 183) or my Berry Cheesecake (page 193).

Bananas are one of the best sources of potassium, which is an essential mineral for maintaining normal blood pressure and a healthy heart. They also have wonderful antacids effects that protect your stomach lining and prevent against ulcers. Plus bananas are a great source of fibre, which – as I'm sure you know by now – is vital for your digestive health and for keeping your blood sugar, and therefore your mood, stable.

BERRIES

I love all types of berries – blueberries, strawberries, raspberries and blackberries. Each one has its own delicious flavour and texture, but they all add a sweet, juicy element to whatever you're cooking. I almost always add berries to my breakfast as I love how much flavour and colour they give whatever I'm eating. They're amazing stirred into my Creamy Coconut Porridge (page 57), scattered over my Sweet Potato Pancakes (page 163) or blended into a smoothie.

Unlike apples and bananas, you can't use berries to stick recipes together. In fact, they actually do the opposite as they make the recipe more watery. So I add them purely for flavour, as in my Apple and Blackberry Crumble (page 189) or my Berry Cheesecake (page 193). The main flavour in both of these are the berries, but all the other ingredients create the structure and textures.

In terms of health benefits, berries are amazing as they're packed with antioxidants, which are so important both for your health and for beautifying your skin and hair, so you'll be glowing from the inside out.

MANGOES

I don't eat mangoes as much as I eat bananas, apple and berries, but I absolutely adore them. They're just so incredibly sweet, juicy and delicious. I love blending them too as they become so insanely creamy when they're blended, as in my Simple Mango and Cashew Mousse (page 184).

As with all fruit, mangoes are packed with fibre, so they'll give you great energy. They're also full of vitamin A, which is important for eye health, as well as vitamin C, which is crucial for a healthy immune system.

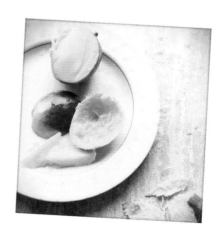

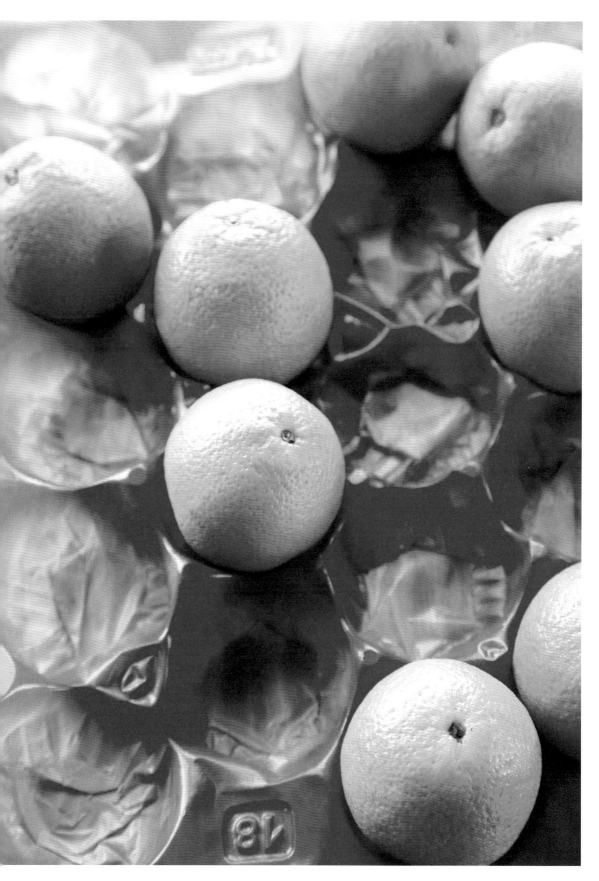

BAKED APPLES *with Coconut Cream*

These baked apples were the last recipe that I did for this book, but they might well be my favourite. Baking the apples with cinnamon, raisins, coconut sugar and pecans means the apple flesh really absorbs all the incredible flavours from each ingredient, so every bite is bursting with flavour. The apples become so soft and tender too when baked, so they really melt in your mouth. The whole thing is then topped with a drizzle of coconut cream, which adds even more flavour and a lovely smooth texture.

Serves 4

For the apples

4 red apples (I use Braeburn apples)
⅔ mug raisins (125g)
2 teaspoons ground cinnamon
2 handfuls of pecans (50g)
5 tablespoons coconut palm sugar

For the coconut cream

100g coconut cream
3 tablespoons date or maple syrup
2 tablespoons coconut palm sugar
2 tablespoons almond butter
 (recipe on page 24)

For the apples

Preheat the oven to 200°C (fan 180°C).

Use an apple corer to take the core out of the apples so that there is a hole from top to bottom.

Mix the raisins, cinnamon, pecans and coconut sugar together.

Place the apples on a baking tray and stuff the core with the raisin mix, then sprinkle all of the leftover mix around the apples.

Drizzle 6 tablespoons water over the leftovers around the apples.

Place the apples in the oven and allow them to bake for 30 minutes, until they're totally soft .

Put each apple in a bowl to serve with a scoop of the raisin mix from the tray, and then pour the coconut cream over everything.

For the coconut cream

Just before the apples finish cooking, make the coconut cream.

Put the coconut cream in a blender with 10 tablespoons boiling water and all the other ingredients and blend until smooth.

Top tip

If you don't have an apple corer, then cut around the core with a knife and scoop out the core with a spoon.

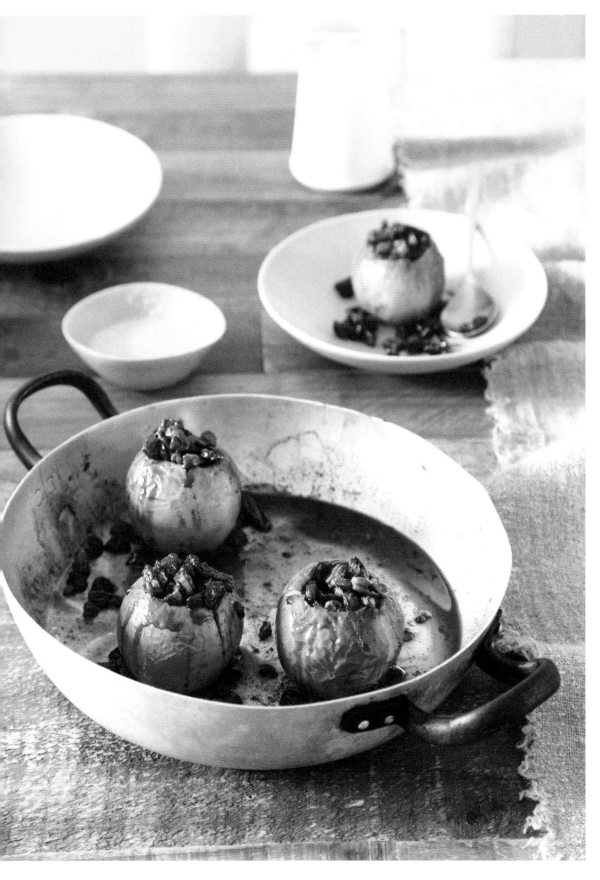

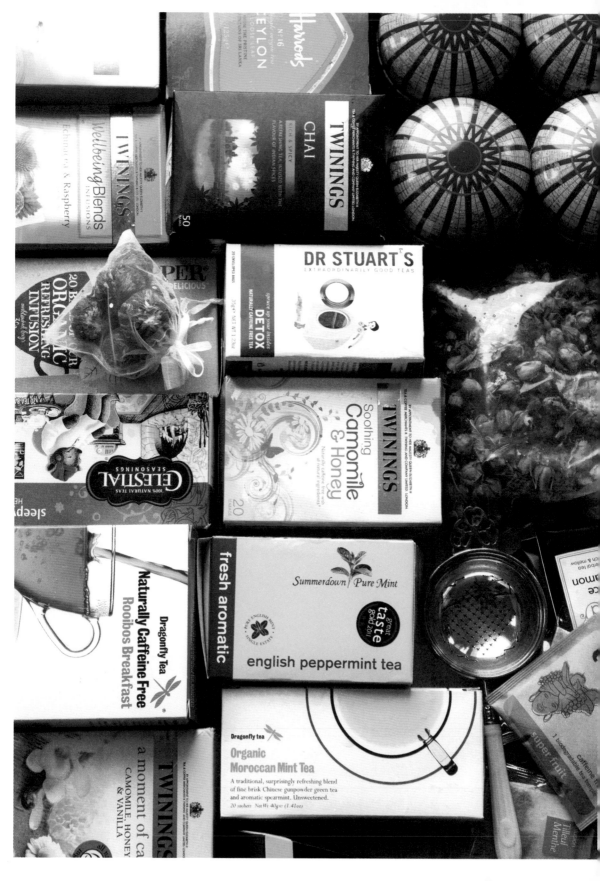

WAFFLES

Everyone loves waffles; they're the happiest breakfast treat! These waffles aren't really so much of a treat though, as they're full of goodness that will really energise your morning, but they still taste incredible. I love eating these with my Date Purée (page 187), a little Strawberry Jam (page 187) and a big mug of herbal tea. You will need a waffle maker to make these though!

makes 8 waffles

3 very ripe large bananas (390g)
4 mugs oat milk (1.2 litres) (recipe on page 20)
3 mugs buckwheat or brown rice flour (600g)
4 tablespoons honey
coconut oil, for greasing

Peel the bananas before placing all the ingredients into a food processor, then blend until the mix is totally smooth.

Grease your waffle maker with coconut oil and allow it to get hot before pouring the mix in.

Allow the mix to cook according to your waffle maker's instructions.

Top tip
Try putting any leftover waffles in the toaster for a minute before you eat them the second time. It makes them extra crispy and delicious.

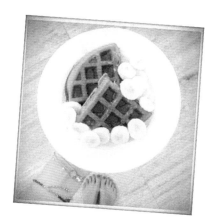

SIMPLE MANGO AND CASHEW MOUSSE

This is one of the easiest recipes in my book. It takes just a couple of minutes to prepare and it always tastes amazing. There's no way that it can go wrong, so you can guarantee that whatever you do, you'll have a great dessert! It's so delicious too and has an especially awesome texture, which is just so thick and creamy. You can eat it as it is or you can add toasted nuts or granola on the top for a little crunch.

Serves 4

4 mangoes (1.2kg)
jar of cashew butter (170g)
8 Medjool dates

Peel the mangoes, then cut the flesh off the stone. I like doing this with a blunt knife as it can be pretty sticky and slippery!

Place the mango into a blender or food processor with the cashew butter and the pitted dates and blend until smooth and creamy.

Pour the mousse into glasses and put them in the fridge for about 30 minutes to set.

Top tip

You can turn this mousse into soft-serve ice cream by slicing the mango and freezing it for about 4 hours before making the dessert. Follow the same instructions as above, but you'll need to do it in a food processor.

BLUEBERRY MUFFINS

These blueberry muffins are unbelievably simple to make and they're a great snack to store in your kitchen to keep you happy and healthy when you're craving something sweet. They're not too sickly either, so you can grab one in the morning for a speedy breakfast on the go.

Makes 12 muffins

2 mugs buckwheat or brown rice
 flour (400g)
1 tablespoon ground cinnamon
1 mug almond milk (300ml)
 (recipe on page 20)
1 mug maple syrup (300ml)
1 mug ground almonds (120g)
3 mugs fresh blueberries (600g)
coconut oil, for greasing

Preheat the oven to 180°C (fan 160°C).

Pour the brown rice, cinnamon, almond milk, maple syrup and ground almonds into a mixing bowl, stirring them to form a smooth batter before adding the blueberries.

Grease a 12-hole muffin tin with the coconut oil, scoop the mixture into it and then bake for about 45 minutes, until the tops begin to turn a golden brown.

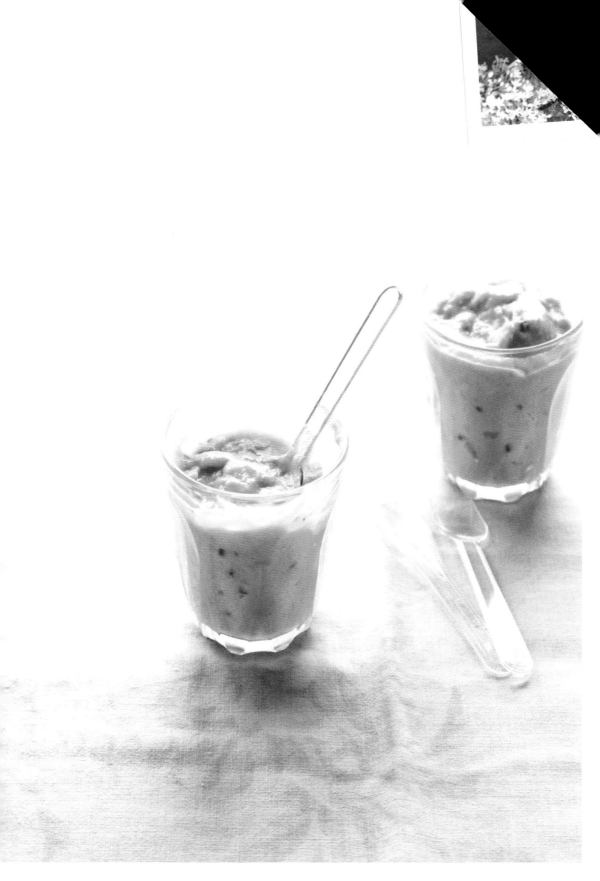

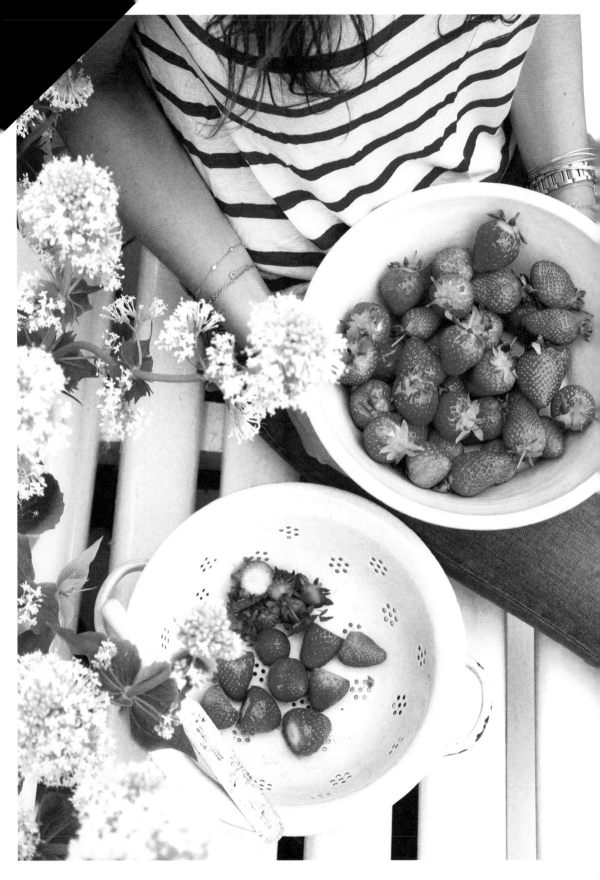

STRAWBERRY JAM

I love jam as it really brightens up breakfast, adding sweet, fruity goodness to whatever you're eating. I love spreading it over slices of my Superfood Bread (page 80), layering it onto my Sweet Potato Pancakes (page 163) and Waffles (page 183) or stirring it into my Creamy Coconut Porridge (page 57). Sadly, most store-brought jams are full of sugar, which is why this version is so amazing – all it contains is 3 tablespoons honey. The magic ingredient here is chia seeds as they thicken up the mixture, giving it the perfect jam consistency.

makes 1 large jar
2 mugs strawberries (400g)
3 tablespoons thick honey
2 tablespoons chia seeds

Chop the green ends off the strawberries and place them in a large saucepan with the honey, turn on the heat and allow them to cook for about 5 minutes until the strawberries are soft.

Mash the strawberries with a potato masher until the mix is quite smooth.

Add in the chia seeds and keep cooking the mix for 20 minutes, on a low heat. Stir every 5 minutes or so.

Remove the pan from the heat and place the jam in a bowl. It will continue to thicken for a few minutes as it cools.

Store the jam in an airtight container in the fridge. It will stay delicious for about a week.

DATE PURÉE

Date purée is one of the most delicious ways to add sweetness to your life. It's a very natural alterative to sugar that can be used on anything from pancakes and waffles to smoothies, toast and porridge. I like to keep a jar in the fridge so that I can add it to my food, knowing that it only contains awesome natural goodness. It also makes a great dip for fruit; try dipping slices of apples and strawberries into a bowl of this – I'm sure you'll love it!

makes 1 large jar
(about 700g)
20 Medjool dates (350g)
optional: 1 teaspoon ground
  cinnamon

Pit the dates, then place them in a blender with 1½ mugs (450ml) water.

Blend at a high speed for a minute or two, until the mix is totally smooth – if you're using cinnamon, then add this now too.

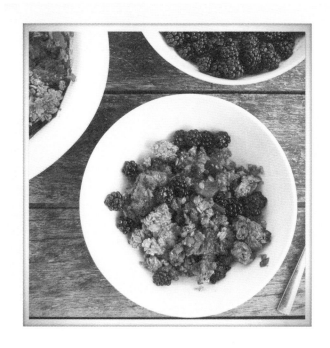

curl up with a bowl of crumble

APPLE AND BLACKBERRY CRUMBLE

Crumble is one of my all-time favourite desserts – it's just divine. Apples and blackberries are one of my best-loved combinations too, especially as they go the most perfect purple colour when baked! I love how the almond, oat and maple topping in this recipe soaks up all the fruity goodness when the crumble bakes, so that every bite is just oozing with juicy goodness. There are hardly any ingredients in this, so you can throw it together really easily and, guess what, they're all amazing for you!

Serves 4

For the topping

1 mug almonds (200g)

1½ mugs oats (180g)

3 heaped tablespoons coconut oil

⅓ mug maple syrup (100ml)

2 teaspoons ground cinnamon

For the fruit layer

6 red apples

2 mugs blackberries (400g)

1 tablespoon maple syrup

1 teaspoon ground cinnamon

For the topping

Start by making the crumble layer. Simply place the almonds in a food processor and blend for a few minutes until a flour forms, then add this flour to a mixing bowl with the oats.

Next, place the coconut oil, maple syrup and cinnamon in a saucepan and gently heat until the coconut has melted and everything has mixed nicely. Pour this over the oat and almond mixture and stir well until all the dry ingredients are coated with the wet ingredients. Leave this bowl to one side.

For the fruit layer

Once you have made the topping, peel the apples and remove the cores, cutting the remaining section into small pieces. Place these in a saucepan with the blackberries, maple syrup and cinnamon and enough boiling water to just cover the bottom of the pan, probably about a centimetre's worth.

Place the lid on the pan and allow it to simmer for about 10 minutes, until the fruit is nice and soft. While this cooks, preheat the oven to 200°C (fan 180°C).

Once the fruit is soft, transfer it to a baking dish and layer the topping above it. Bake for 25–30 minutes, until the top is nicely browned. Serve and enjoy!

Top tip

Try eating the leftovers of the crumble for breakfast with a little coconut yoghurt or almond milk – it's so delicious!

BAKED BANANAS

Stuffed with melted Dark Chocolate

These baked bananas were one of my favourite foods growing up. We used to stuff them with chopped-up pieces of Mars Bars and a little golden syrup, so not exactly the same as this version, which uses dark chocolate, cinnamon and dates. However, both taste as good as each other, and this version makes you feel a million times better, so it's absolutely the winner!

Serves 4

4 very ripe bananas

1 teaspoon ground cinnamon

4 Medjool dates

60g chocolate (I use raw chocolate, which only uses coconut sugar,
　　but dark chocolate works too)

Preheat the oven to 200°C (fan 180°C).

Slice each banana in half without going all the way to the bottom, so that they're still whole. Place each banana on its own sheet of tin foil, which needs to be big enough to totally wrap around it and seal it.

Sprinkle the cinnamon into the split of the four bananas, sharing it evenly among them.

Remove the stones and cut up the dates, then put the pieces on top of the cinnamon.

Finally, break up the chocolate and spread it evenly on top of the dates.

Wrap the foil around each banana and bake for 10 minutes until the chocolate has melted and the bananas are deliciously soft.

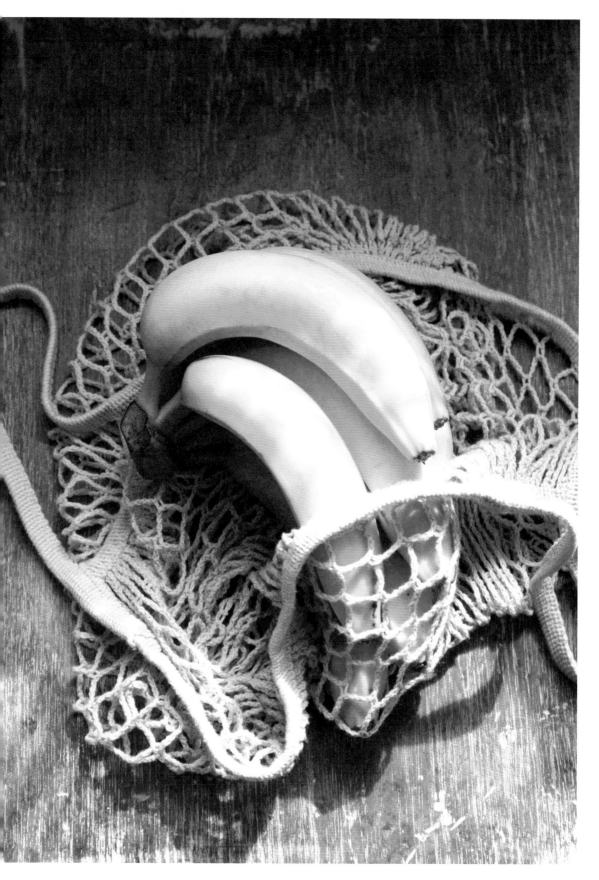

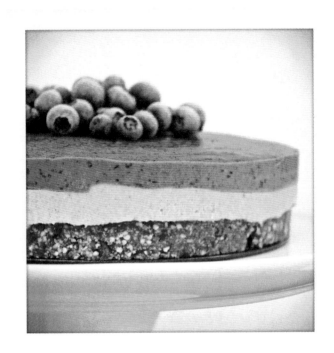

perfection...

BERRY CHEESECAKE

This is one of my most popular recipes on the blog; I think this is partly because it's so beautiful! The three layers really look amazing next to each other and, more importantly, they taste incredible too. The base is a sticky date and almond biscuit; the middle is a smooth, thick blend of sweet cashews, banana, maple syrup and apple juice; and the top is a creamy berry mix with juicy blueberries and strawberries.

Makes 12–15 slices

For the base
1½ mugs almonds (300g)
2½ mugs Medjool dates (500g)

For the middle layer
2 over-ripe bananas
2 mugs cashew nuts (400g)
½ mug maple syrup (150ml)
⅓ mug fresh apple juice (100ml)
1 teaspoon ground cinnamon

For the top layer
1 banana
1 mug fresh blueberries (200g)
1 mug strawberries (200g)
4 Medjool dates
1 tablespoon maple syrup
1 teaspoon ground cinnamon

Before making this, you need to slice the three bananas and freeze the slices for at least 3 hours along with the blueberries (packaged frozen berries have too high a water content and make the mix too runny, so you need to freeze your own). You also need to soak the cashew nuts for at least 3 hours in a bowl of water.

For the base
Once you're ready to start cooking, begin with the base. Place the almonds into a food processor and blend for a minute or so until the nuts are nicely crushed. Then add the pitted Medjool dates and blend again until a sticky mix forms. Press this into the base of a cake tin and place in the freezer.

For the middle layer
Next, make the middle layer by simply putting all the ingredients into the food processor and blending until smooth and creamy. Take the base layer out of the freezer and pour three-quarters of this mix over it before putting the cake back into the freezer. Keep the final quarter of the mix in the processor as it's needed for the top layer.

For the top layer
Wait about 20 minutes for the middle layer to set in the freezer before making the third layer. To make this, simply add the remaining ingredients to the blender with the last of the mix from the middle, then blend until smooth and pour over the middle layer.

Place the cake back into the freezer to set for 2–3 hours before serving. You'll need to remove the cake from the freezer and allow it to warm up for a few minutes before you serve it.

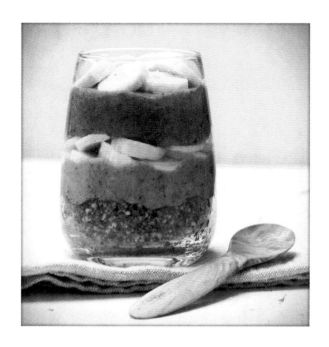

hard to believe this is healthy!

BANOFFEE PIE

This is another favourite recipe from the blog and it's my friends' and family's favourite too – none of us can get enough of it! The best thing about this Banoffee Pie is that not one bite of it tastes healthy, in fact it tastes the total opposite – rich, creamy, sweet and decadent, which is awesome as all the ingredients are so nourishing. I promise that this really is so much better than the traditional recipe!

Serves 2

For the first layer

½ mug pecans (70g)

½ mug almonds (100g)

2 teaspoons almond butter (recipe on page 24)

2 tablespoons raw honey (maple syrup also works)

2 Medjool dates

For the middle layer

2 very ripe bananas

2 tablespoons almond butter (recipe on page 24)

For the top layer

6 Medjool dates, pitted

4 tablespoons almond butter (recipe on page 24)

1 over-ripe banana, plus 1 more banana for layering

For the first layer

Start by making the base. Place the nuts in a food processor and blend for a minute or two until a crumbly mix forms, then add the almond butter, honey and dates and blend again. Once it's nice and sticky, stop blending and fill the bottom of two glasses with the nutty goodness, pressing it down firmly with a spoon to set.

For the middle layer

Next, make the banana cream layer by simply placing the bananas and almond butter in the processor and blending until smooth. Put this on top of the nutty layer and place in the freezer for 20 minutes to set.

For the top layer

While this freezes, make the caramel layer by simply placing all its ingredients into the food processor with 4 tablespoons water and blending again until smooth.

After 20 minutes, remove the glasses from the freezer and slice the final banana in layers over the banana cream before adding the caramel layer.

Top tip

I like serving this in glasses as individual little pies, but it works great in a cake tin too as a whole pie.

KEY LIME PIE

This Key Lime Pie is one of the more adventurous recipes in the book and I'm sure that as you look at the ingredients list, you'll be questioning whether or not it really does taste good; so you're going to have to trust me that it does taste wonderful. The avocado and coconut milk together make the dessert insanely creamy, while the lime gives it a fantastically fresh flavour and the maple syrup adds some delicious sweetness. Don't worry, you can't taste the avocado in it at all!

Serves 10–12

For the base
2 mugs almonds (400g)
about 30 Medjool dates (600g),
    pitted
2 tablespoons coconut oil

For the middle
5 very ripe avocados
juice of 3 limes (30ml)
¾ mug maple syrup (225ml)
4 tablespoons coconut milk (I
    take the tablespoons from the
    solid part of the milk in the
    tin, not the liquid part)
1 more lime, to grate

For the base
Start by making the base. Place the almonds into a food processor and blend for a minute or so until they break down into pieces (not as smooth as a flour though).

Add the dates to the food processor with the coconut oil and blend again, until the dates have all been crushed and the mix is sticky.

Use a spatula to press the almond and date mix firmly into a 20–25cm cake tin – the base should be about 2–3cm thick and very compact. Leave the base to one side while you make the middle.

For the middle
Scoop the flesh out of the avocados, discarding the stones, and place all the flesh into your food processor. Add in the lime juice, maple syrup and coconut milk and blend until the mix is totally smooth and creamy.

Pour the mix onto the base and place the cake tin in the freezer to set for about an hour and a half – you want it to be firm but not frozen!

Once you're ready to serve, grate the zest of the remaining lime over the top of the pie.

Top tip
Make sure that the flesh of your avocados is really green. If they have brown spots in them, then your pie will look less vibrant green and more swamp colour!

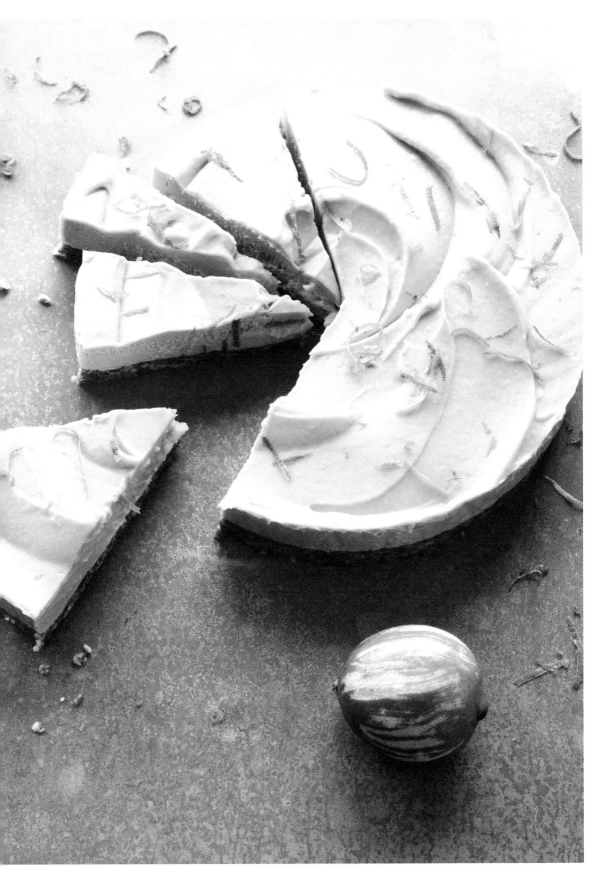

BANANA ICE CREAM

One-ingredient banana ice cream is the most magical recipe I've ever created. Honestly, the first time I made it I was dancing around my kitchen, literally, singing with happiness because this really does taste identical to ice cream. In fact, it may even be more delicious as it has a smoother, creamier texture. I know it's hard to believe that frozen bananas can make ice cream without even having to use an ice-cream maker, but trust me on this one – you'll love it! I love making the classic version, but you can spice it up too and add frozen berries to make a berry flavour, or dates and almond butter to make a caramel version.

Serves 4

FOR THE CLASSIC VERSION

8 very ripe large bananas (1.3kg)

FOR THE BERRY VERSION

½ mug frozen blueberries or mixed frozen berries (100g)

FOR THE CARAMEL VERSION

12 Medjool dates, pitted

5 tablespoons almond butter (recipe page 24)

Peel the bananas, then chop them into thin slices.

Place the slices in a bowl in the freezer for at least 6 hours.

Once you're ready to make your ice cream, remove the banana slices from the freezer and allow them to warm up for 5 minutes or so.

Place the slices in a food processor and blend for a minute or two, until the mix is totally smooth and delicious. At this point, add the frozen berries or dates and almond butter if you're using them and blend.

Top tip

Let your bananas go really over-ripe before you freeze them – it'll make the ice cream much smoother. This is a great way to use up old bananas too as they can stay frozen for weeks, so they'll be waiting for you when the ice cream cravings strike!

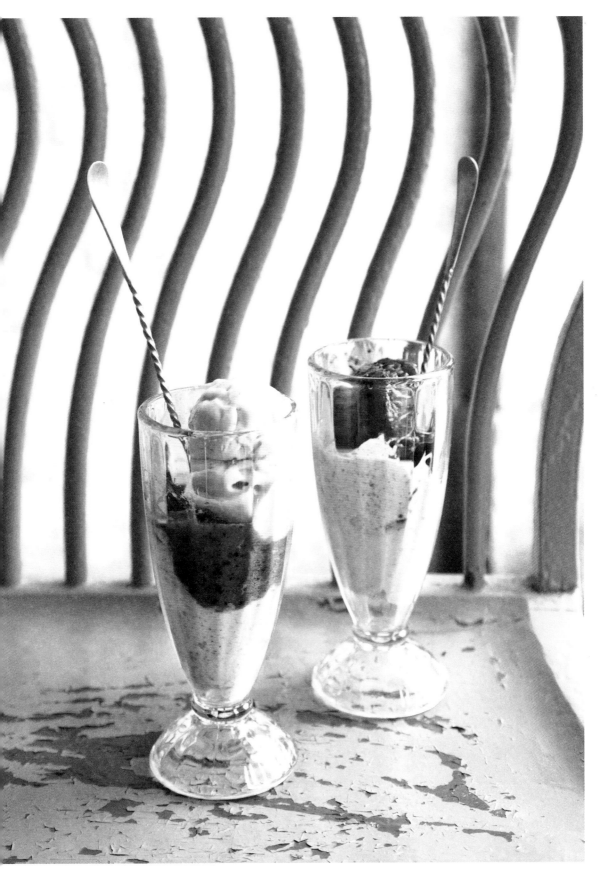

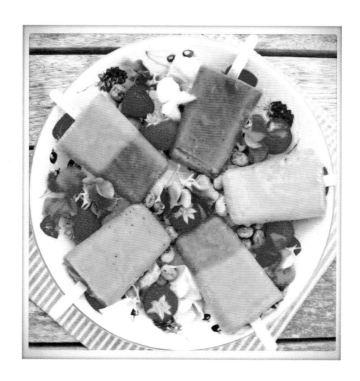

chill out

ICE LOLLIES

These ice lollies are one of my favourite recipes from my blog. They just take a couple of minutes to make and they last for ages in the freezer, so you have something amazing to snack on at all times during the summer. All three flavours – chocolate, strawberry and banana cinnamon – are made from a base of coconut milk to create a perfectly creamy texture, while the dates make them perfectly sweet.

makes 2 of each flavour (6 lollies in total)

CHOCOLATE

2 Medjool dates
2 ripe bananas
1 heaped teaspoon raw cacao powder
2 tablespoons coconut milk

STRAWBERRY

2 Medjool dates
1 ripe banana
1 mug strawberries (200g)
2 tablespoons coconut milk

BANANA CINNAMON

2 Medjool dates
2 ripe bananas
1 teaspoon ground cinnamon
2 tablespoons coconut milk

Simply remove the stones from the dates and peel the bananas. Then place the ingredients for your chosen flavour into a blender with 2 tablespoons water and blend for a minute until smooth.

Pour into an ice-lolly mould and freeze, doing the same for each flavour. To make mixed ones, simply pour half of one flavour into a mould, allow it to freeze for an hour, and then top the mould up with the second flavour.

The lollies need to freeze for about 5 hours before they are ready to be enjoyed!

Top tip

Try switching up the ingredients in these. Always keep the coconut milk and water as your base, but then try adding things like mango and pineapple for new flavours.

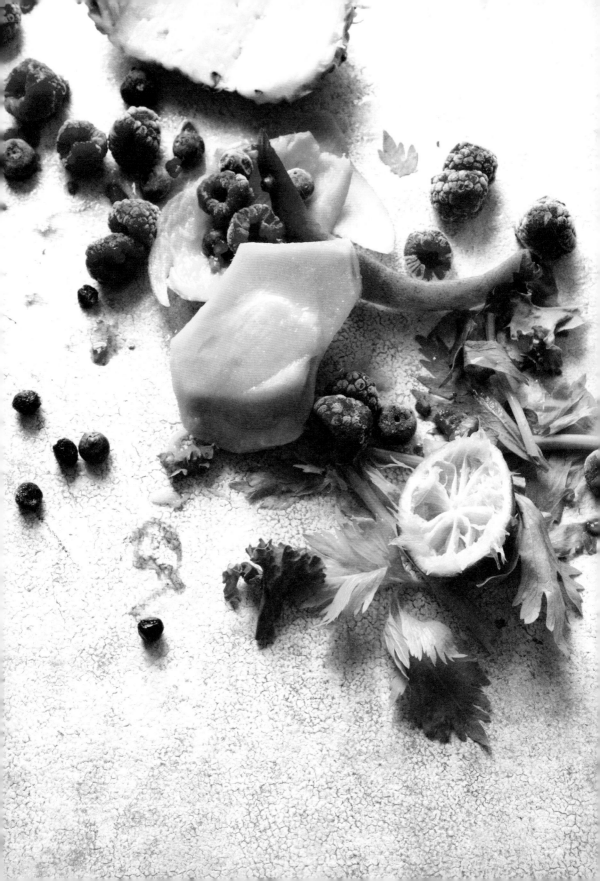

SMOOTHIES AND JUICES

blended to perfection

GREEN GODDESS SMOOTHIE

TROPICAL MANGO, PINEAPPLE AND COCONUT SMOOTHIE

CLASSIC BERRY SMOOTHIE

BEST BREAKFAST SMOOTHIE

SIMPLE BANANA AND SPINACH SMOOTHIE

OATY SMOOTHIE

PEAR, POMEGRANATE AND BASIL SMOOTHIE

MANGO, KIWI AND GINGER SMOOTHIE

ACAI BOWL

MINT CHOCOLATE MILKSHAKE

BANANA MILKSHAKE

CARROT, APPLE AND GINGER JUICE

CUCUMBER, PEAR AND MINT JUICE

BEETROOT JUICE

GLOWING GREEN JUICE

WATERMELON, CUCUMBER AND MINT JUICE

PINEAPPLE, CUCUMBER AND GINGER JUICE

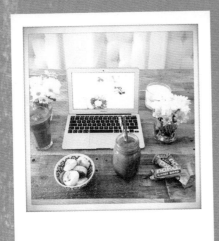

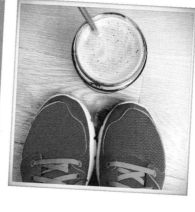

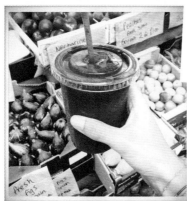

'Reading your story was like a light bulb moment for me. I will never look back. I was inspired to take on the vegan lifestyle and I can honestly say I have noticed the biggest change in my health.' — Sarah

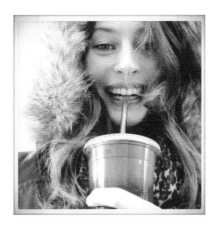

smoothies and juices

I'm obsessed with both smoothies and juices and both have played a huge part in my healing journey. I start every day with one or the other and now seem to be a total addict! There are so many reasons why I love them. Of course the fact that they taste so amazing is the main reason, but beyond that I find that drinking a big glass of goodness first thing in the morning really does wonders for your mental and physical health.

Mentally there's something really empowering about making a conscious decision to start your day by doing something so nourishing and nurturing for yourself before you've made any other decisions; it really puts you on the right track to have a positive day. Of course, for your body it's incredible too, as you get such a wonderful array of vitamins and minerals in each glass so you'll feel incredibly energised and ready for anything! Try having a smoothie or a glass of juice every morning for a week and see how you feel – I can guarantee that you'll feel better than ever.

So what's the difference between a juice and a smoothie? Juices need a juicer to make and

contain no fibre – it's all taken out by the juicer so you're left with pure juice. This means that juices aren't as filling as smoothies, so if I have a juice for breakfast, I'll eat something with it, normally a bowl of Granola (page 76) with Almond Milk (page 24) and fresh fruit, a few slices of my Superfood Bread (page 80) with mashed avocado or a bowl of my Creamy Coconut Porridge (page 57). Juices take a little longer to make than smoothies and require more washing up, but on the plus side a juice gives you more goodness much quicker as there is no fibre, so the vitamins are absorbed straight into the bloodstream. This does mean though that we need to watch the sugar intake of the juice as there's no fibre to cushion it, which is why we add some green veggies to each one or drink it with a meal.

Smoothies, on the other hand, are made in a blender and retain all the original fibre of whatever you're blending. This means that the smoothie is much more filling. So if I make a smoothie for breakfast, I'll have just that, as I fill it with a little of everything to make sure I've got lots of great plant protein, fats and vitamins to keep me happily full until lunchtime. Smoothies are much quicker to make too. It takes me less than five minutes to make one and clean the blender – and then you can just take it on the go with you for a speedy breakfast.

There are some fruits and veggies that work better in a juice and others that work better in a smoothie; it really depends on their water content. In general, the higher the water content of your fruit and vegetable, the better it is in a juice – so cucumbers, celery, apples, carrots, fennel and pineapple all juice really well, whereas you'll find mangoes, bananas, spinach, avocados and pears all blend well and are therefore better in smoothies – they don't really give you much juice if you juice them. Lots of people juice leafy greens, like spinach and kale too, but I don't love doing that because you need such a crazy amount of each to get such a small amount of juice that I find it's a waste. Instead I'll make my juice and then put it in the blender with the spinach or kale or I'll just make a smoothie with them.

In terms of storing smoothies and juices, you can make them in advance, but you then need to keep them in airtight containers in the fridge. I find that they stay fresh for about three days in the fridge after you've made them, so you can make enough for three days in one sitting. If I want to make a couple of portions of a drink though, then they do need to be stored in separate containers as once you open them, you should ideally drink them within a few hours if you want to get maximum goodness from them. I keep mine in recycled glass jars, which look pretty and means that they're very portable as they have lids.

Over the next few pages I've shared lots of my favourite recipes for both smoothies and juices, but I also want to help you learn how to build them yourself. They're actually unbelievably easy – you just need a few simple building blocks and then you can get really creative with your combinations!

HOW TO MAKE A SMOOTHIE

Steps one and two are the most important – you can't make a smoothie without them – the other steps are all optional though, so you can then pick and choose from them. I normally add something from each step, but you absolutely don't have to.

1 Pick a liquid. I use one of the following for each smoothie: water, coconut water, almond milk, oat milk, rice milk, coconut milk or the juice of a cucumber. The amount of each you use is totally up to you. I like my smoothies really thick so am quite sparing with my liquid, but if you like them runnier, then add a little more. If you're after something cold, then add a few ice cubes too.

2 Choose a base. The base needs to be a chunky fruit or vegetable – normally avocado, mango or banana. These all ensure that the smoothie is deliciously thick and creamy. You really need to have at least one of the three. If you want something incredibly creamy, then use a mix of two. Banana is my go-to as it works in absolutely any flavour combination, but they're all delicious.

3 Add a second or third fruit for flavour. For this I normally add berries (frozen or fresh), pineapple, pear, kiwi or papaya, as these all blend really well and add a delicious flavour without making it too thick.

4 Add some exciting extras to bulk it out. If I make a smoothie for breakfast I like it to be really filling, so I add ingredients like nut butter (almond butter is my favourite), porridge oats, soaked nuts, hemp protein powder or coconut yoghurt. All of these are filled with either plant protein or fibre, so they help to keep you energised for hours, while also adding extra creaminess.

5 Mix in some superfoods. Spirulina, maca, baobab, acai, cacao, chia seeds, hemp protein and chlorella are all incredible. I mix and match them depending on what I feel my body needs that day. I have spirulina every day though, as it's great for plant protein and for B12. Have a look at the Superfoods section (below) to see what the benefits

of each of them are and when's best to use them.

6 Sweeten it up a little. If you'd like to sweeten your smoothie up, then add a couple of pitted Medjool dates, some raw honey or a dash of maple syrup. The quantity of each is pretty dependent on your own taste buds, so start with one date or a teaspoon of sweetener and go from there until you reach your perfect sweetness.

7 Finally, sneak in some greens. Spinach is my favourite green for smoothies as it blends really easily and changes the colour of the smoothie without changing the taste. Kale is much stronger in flavour and doesn't blend as easily so I'd only use it if you're a smoothie connoisseur and you have a really strong blender, otherwise you'll be sipping on lumps of kale!

8 Blend everything together, sip and feel instantly healthier!

HOW TO MAKE A JUICE

Making a juice is simpler in some ways, but it's slower and requires more washing up! The plus side is that you get more goodness much quicker as there is no fibre, so the vitamins are absorbed straight into the bloodstream. As there's no fibre, it's good to make sure it includes some greens to decrease the sugar content.

1 Pick two bases: cucumbers, celery, apples, carrots, fennel and pineapple work best as they're the juiciest, so will give you the most liquid.

2 Add a couple of other fruits or veggies. These can be a little more fibrous, but they do still need to be quite juicy and not overly fleshy like bananas, mangoes or avocados. I normally use beetroot, pears, kiwis, strawberries, melon, broccoli, oranges or grapefruit, which all work amazingly well.

3 Add a kick. To create a bit more depth to your juice, add 2–3cm ginger, the juice of half a lemon or a lime.

4 Get some cleaning greens in. To get some extra green cleansing benefits, you can also add a small handful of parsley, mint, coriander or basil to the juicer. In order to get the most from these, add them at the same time as your base.

5 Add some fibre. If you'd like to add some fibre to your juice, then stir in a tablespoon of something fibrous like wheatgrass. You won't taste it, but it will slow down the absorption of the juice. This is really awesome as it will mean the juice keeps you energised for longer, and if it's quite a fruity juice, it will help cushion the sugar.

6 Blend in some greens. As I said above, I don't love juicing spinach or kale, so once I've made the juice, I pour it into my blender with a handful of one or the other and then blend until it's nice and smooth.

SUPERFOODS

The last thing I want to talk about before we get into the recipes are superfoods. I know that the word superfood is a pretty broad description for something and it can really be applied to so many things, from spinach to quinoa, bananas to avocados, but it's also often used specifically to talk about all the different powders that you can add to your smoothies.

There are so many of them, but the most common are spirulina, maca, wheatgrass, baobab, acai and hemp. None of them are essential in any of the recipes, and you can absolutely leave them out. I do use them a lot though and find they do wonders for my health, so I wanted to share a little information on each one with you.

All these superfoods can be found in health-food shops, online and they're even stocked on websites like Amazon!

SPIRULINA

Spirulina is my go-to superfood and I use it every day. It comes in powder form and has a really strong taste, which you learn to love, but start small to get used to it. I'd recommend just half a teaspoon for the first week or so and then build

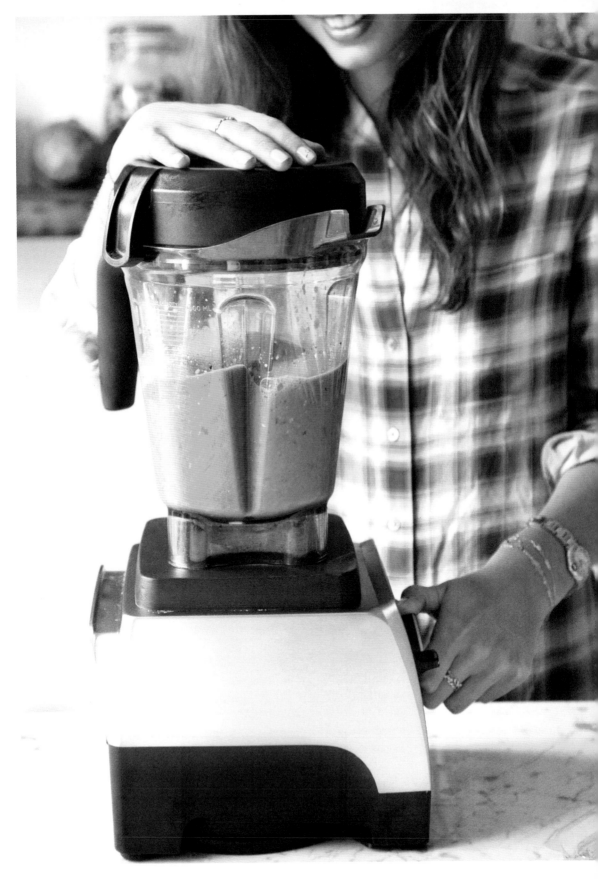

up. So what is spirulina and why take it when it tastes weird? Spirulina is a freshwater algae, which is made up of around sixty to seventy per cent complete proteins. This means that it's incredibly energising and helps to keep your blood sugar balanced, which keeps your happiness balanced too! The protein is also incredibly easy for your body to break down, much easier than any animal source. It's also like taking a serious multivitamin as it's bursting with iron, calcium, magnesium, vitamin E, selenium, zinc, B vitamins and many others.

MACA

Maca has a pretty cool history: it originates from a root in South America, and the story goes that the Inca warriors used to take it before going into battle to increase their strength and stamina! Whilst this is really funny, it actually makes sense as maca contains unique energy-boosting compounds called macamides and macaenes, so taking it really does boost your energy. Its other incredible property is its ability to stabilise and regulate our hormone levels, helping us to feel more balanced. It doesn't have a strong flavour and if anything it tastes a little like caramel, so the powder blends into smoothies really nicely and leaves the original flavour pretty much unchanged. This means it's much easier to use than something like spirulina.

WHEATGRASS

I have to be honest and admit that wheatgrass is my least favourite of all the superfoods. I know it's really good for me, but I'm not obsessed with the taste. The reason it's so good (and why I should learn to love it), is because it's bursting with chlorophyll and antioxidants. It's also filled with amazing amounts of fibre and vitamin A, which are really important for glowing skin and strong, shiny hair. It just tastes quite grassy, but once you get past that, it will do incredible things for you. You can buy wheatgrass shots from juice bars, which come in liquid form, but in my smoothies I use wheatgrass powder.

ACAI

Acai, on the other hand, is the most delicious of all the superfoods. It tastes like a very rich berry, so it's amazing in any berry-oriented smoothie as it really intensifies all the awesome original flavours. You can buy it either as a powder, which I normally do, or as a frozen purée. It comes from the acai berry in Brazil and it's famous for being unbelievably rich in antioxidants – better than blueberries even! It's also packed with vitamin E, which is so important for beautiful skin, as well as lots of essential fatty acids.

BAOBAB

After acai, baobab is my favourite superfood as it's also really delicious. It has a more subtle flavour than acai, and seems to just taste generally sweet and fruity. It originates from the beautiful baobab tree in Africa and it's famed for its immune boosting properties as it's so rich in vitamin C. It actually contains about six times more vitamin C than oranges gram per gram, so I use it for a few days whenever I'm feeling run down and it instantly picks me back up again. It's also full of iron, which is amazing for boosting your energy levels.

HEMP

Hemp powder is a wonderful source of protein. I know people think that vegans/vegetarians must struggle to get protein, but it's pretty easy once you know where to look and something like hemp is a great start. I add a tablespoon or two, alongside spirulina and nut butter, to my smoothie every morning to energise me for the day. It's really important not to skimp on protein too, as it is so important for both your energy and your mood. Hemp is a fantastic protein source as it's a complete protein, so contains all the essential amino acids, as well as a whole host of other awesome vitamins and minerals.

So let's get blending and juicing!

EIGHT DELICIOUS SMOOTHIES

My first smoothie will make you feel like a goddess – it's so healing and I'm really grateful to it for giving me so much energy over the last few years! It is a very green smoothie though, so you could replace the avocado with banana to make it a little sweeter. If you're new to smoothies, then the berry smoothie is a great place to start as it looks beautiful and tastes like dessert! The tropical smoothie just tastes like summer! I love having it for breakfast, adding oats to make it more filling.

makes 1 large glass

GREEN GODDESS SMOOTHIE

3 stalks of celery

1 apple

1 cucumber

2-3cm piece of fresh ginger

1 small ripe avocado

optional: 1 teaspoon spirulina

1 heaped teaspoon almond butter (recipe
   on page 24)

4 big stalks of kale

Put the celery, apple, cucumber and ginger through a juicer and collect the juice.

Put the juice into a blender with the flesh of the avocado, the spirulina, if using, and the almond butter. Tear the kale leaves off their stems and add them to the blender too. Blend at a high speed until perfectly smooth.

TROPICAL MANGO, PINEAPPLE AND COCONUT SMOOTHIE

½ mango (150g)

thick slice of pineapple (200g)

1 mug coconut water (300ml)

handful of cashew nuts

2 tablespoons coconut milk

juice of ½ lime

optional: handful of porridge oats

Peel the mango using a vegetable peeler and cut its flesh off the stone into the blender. Add the remaining ingredients and blend until smooth and creamy.

CLASSIC BERRY SMOOTHIE

1 ripe banana

⅓ mug raspberries (70g)

⅓ mug blueberries (70g)

⅓ mug strawberries (70g)

3 tablespoons coconut milk

1 teaspoon almond butter (recipe on page 24)

Simply peel the banana, then place it in a blender with the berries, coconut milk and almond butter and blend until smooth and creamy.

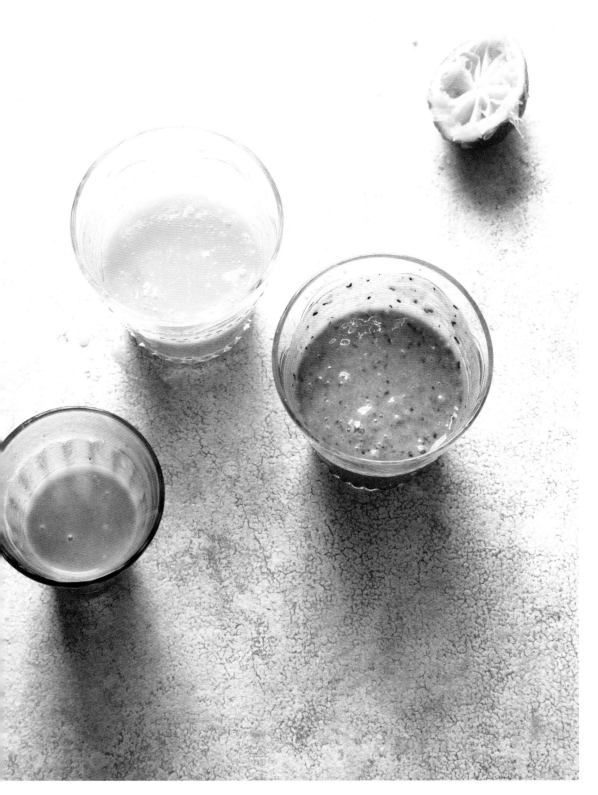

My breakfast smoothie gives you all the energy you need to have a great day, while this oat smoothie is incredibly soothing and is my favourite late-night snack. The banana and spinach smoothie is the best green smoothie for beginners. It looks green and you get lots of green goodness from the spinach, but crucially it doesn't taste green. It will gently introduce you to the concept of drinking veggies before you transition to greener drinks.

Makes 1 large glass

BEST BREAKFAST SMOOTHIE

½ ripe avocado
1 ripe banana, peeled
1 mug cold almond milk (300ml) (recipe
   on page 20)
½ mug frozen berries (100g)
¼ mug oats (30g)
handful of spinach
optional: 2 Medjool dates, pitted

Scoop the avocado flesh out of its skin, discarding the stone. Place everything into a blender and blend until smooth and creamy.

SIMPLE BANANA AND SPINACH SMOOTHIE

1 ripe banana, peeled
big handful of spinach
2 Medjool dates, pitted
1 heaped teaspoon almond butter (recipe
   on page 24)
½ mug cold water or almond milk (150ml)
   (recipe on page 20)

Place all the ingredients into your blender and blend until smooth. If you like your smoothie runnier, add a little more water.

OATY SMOOTHIE

4 brazil nuts
1½ mugs oats (180g)
1 ripe banana, peeled
2 Medjool dates, pitted
1 heaped teaspoon ground cinnamon
1 teaspoon honey
optional superfoods: 1 teaspoon maca and/
   or 1 teaspoon baobab powder

Leave the brazil nuts and oats to soak in a bowl of cold water for an hour or so to soften, or overnight.

Drain the water from the oats and nuts and then place them in a blender with the peeled banana, pitted dates, cinnamon, honey, maca and/or baobab powders, if using, and ½ mug (150ml) fresh water. Blend until smooth and creamy.

These two fruit smoothies are soothing, unbelievably refreshing and work perfectly on a hot day. Try freezing them in ice lolly moulds. The flavours are so strong that they make the best ice lollies!

Makes 1 large or 2 small glasses

PEAR, POMEGRANATE AND BASIL SMOOTHIE

1 ripe banana

1 pear

1 mug cold almond milk (300ml)
   (recipe on page 20)

⅓ mug pomegranate seeds (80g)

handful of raspberries (40g)

handful of fresh basil leaves

1 tablespoon almond butter
   (recipe on page 24)

Simply peel the banana and peel and core the pear, and then place all of the ingredients into a blender and blend until smooth and creamy.

MANGO, KIWI AND GINGER SMOOTHIE

½ mango (150g)

1cm piece of fresh ginger

1 kiwi

½ mug frozen berries (100g)

¾ mug cold coconut water or almond/oat
   milk (225ml) (recipe on page 20)

juice of ½ lime

Peel the mango using a vegetable peeler and cut its flesh off the stone. Peel the ginger using the vegetable peeler. Scoop the kiwi flesh out of its skin.

Place everything in a blender and blend until smooth.

ACAI BOWL

This honestly tastes more like dessert than a smoothie; it's similar to ice cream, but more flavoursome. I really think it's the sweetest, creamiest, most delicious bowl of goodness you'll ever eat. I love piling my Acai Bowl high with lots of Cinnamon Pecan Granola (page 76) plus some fresh fruit and a generous dollop of coconut yoghurt!

Serves 1

1 packet of frozen acai (100g)

1 ripe banana

2 Medjool dates

1 tablespoon almond butter (recipe on
   page 24)

½ mug frozen blueberries (100g)

Place the acai packet in a mug of boiling water for about 20 seconds, then once it's starting to melt, remove the packet from the mug, cut it open and pour the contents into a blender.

Peel the banana and pit the dates, then add them to the blender along with the almond butter and frozen blueberries. Finally, blend until everything is smooth and creamy.

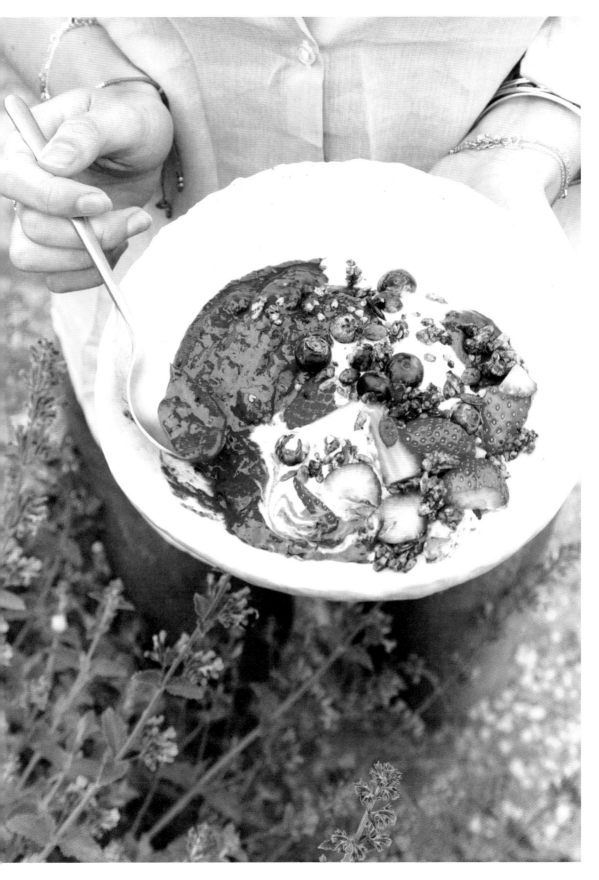

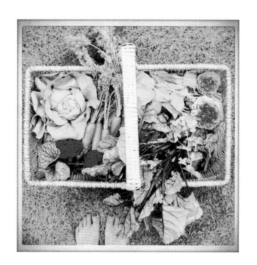

'I've had a terrible 6 months and have been really down and sad most days. I came across your blog and decided to try out the hummus and all I can say is, your food has lifted me out of an extremely dark hole. Thank you so very much for your blog, it's amazing, the food is so delicious and healthy and it has turned my life around' – Rosie

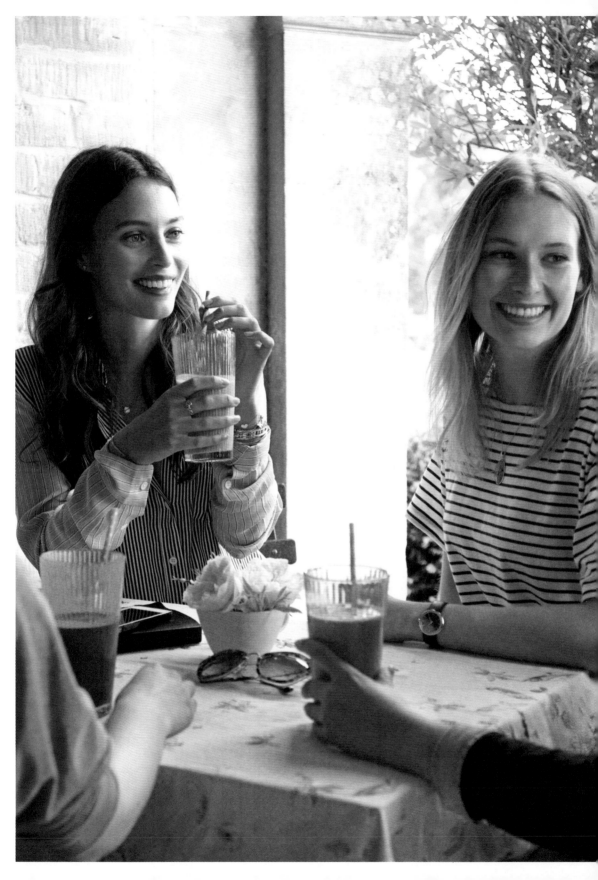

MINT CHOCOLATE MILKSHAKE

This milkshake is even better then it sounds – it's just so unbelievably rich, smooth and creamy. It tastes totally unhealthy even though it's actually packed with goodness, which I love as it means that you can enjoy a milkshake for breakfast and feel great about it!

makes 1 large glass

small handful of fresh mint

½ ripe avocado

1 ripe banana, peeled

1 mug cold almond milk
   (300ml) (recipe on page 20)

3 Medjool dates, pitted

2 teaspoons raw cacao powder

Pull the mint leaves off their sprigs and scoop the avocado flesh out of the skin and remove the stone.

Place all the ingredients into a blender and blend until smooth and creamy.

Top tip

Try adding half the amount of almond milk, so that it's really thick, and then pour granola over it for the best breakfast ever.

BANANA MILKSHAKE

This tastes just like a caramel milkshake – it's pretty awesome. The combination of dates, almond butter, banana and cinnamon is totally magical. As with the chocolate milkshake, it's really hard to believe that this is healthy, but it really is so nutritious and energising, so now you can enjoy milkshakes in the knowledge that each delicious sip is doing amazing things for you.

Serves 1

1 large ripe banana

3 Medjool dates

¾ mug cold almond milk
   (300ml) (recipe on page 20)

1 tablespoon almond butter
   (recipe on page 20)

1 teaspoon ground cinnamon

optional: 2 teaspoons maca

Peel the bananas and remove the stones from the dates.

Place all the ingredients in a blender and blend until smooth. If you'd like it to be runnier, then you can add more almond milk or water at this point.

Top tip

Try using frozen slices of banana to make this even thicker and more ice-cream-like.

SIX AMAZING JUICES

The mint in this cucumber juice is very soothing and particularly great at calming your digestive system and relieving nausea, so it's a perfect juice to pick you up if you're feeling unwell. The pulp from this carrot juice is my favourite one to use in the Superfood Crackers (page 82), so don't throw it away after you've juiced. The beetroot juice is pretty veggie-heavy, but beetroot actually has a really sweet flavour that combines well with the apple to cut the savoury nature of the other veggies.

makes 1 large glass

CARROT, APPLE AND GINGER JUICE

1cm piece of fresh ginger
3 medium red apples
4 large carrots

Put the ginger into the juicer at the beginning with a piece of apple to get the most flavour from it. Then simply put everything through the juicer and collect the juice.

CUCUMBER, PEAR AND MINT JUICE

large handful of fresh mint leaves
1 cucumber
2 apples
2 pears

Juice the mint leaves at the beginning with either the cucumber or an apple. Doing this will allow you to get more flavour from the mint leaves. Then simply place all of the ingredients into your juicer and watch the deliciousness pour out.

BEETROOT JUICE

1cm piece of fresh ginger
1 medium red apple
1 medium beetroot
1 small cucumber
1 small fennel bulb
2 large carrots

Peel the skin off the beetroot (keeping it on makes the juice too earthy for my liking). Put everything through the juicer. I like to add the ginger at the beginning with the apple to get maximum flavour from it.

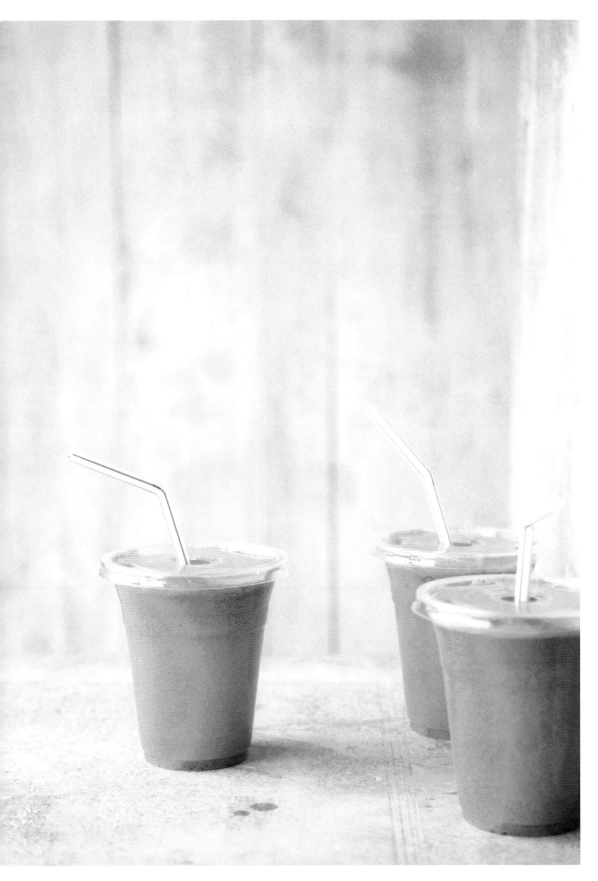

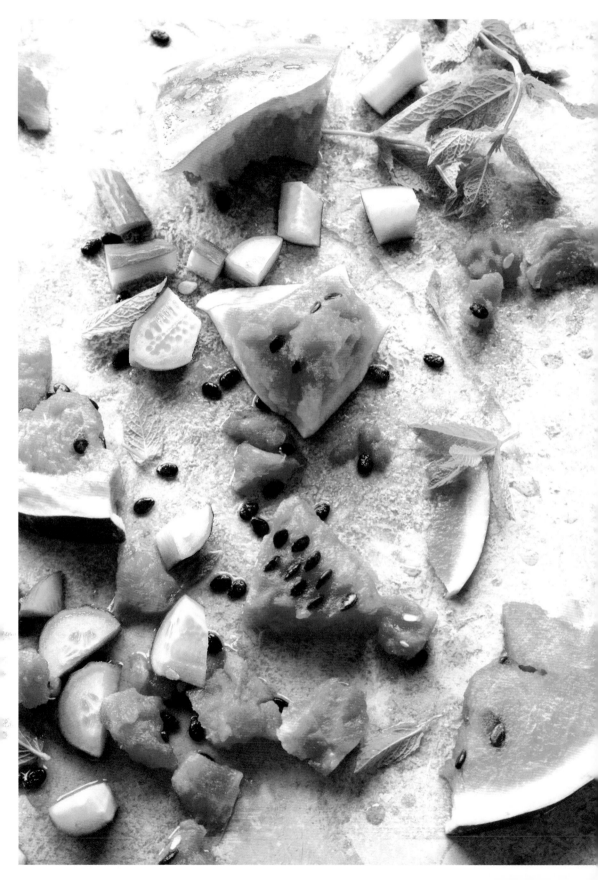

Green juice is one of the most healing things on the planet. The greener the juice (and this Glowing Green Juice is a very green juice), the better it is for us as there's more chlorophyll, which works to alkalinise your body, detox and purify it and boost your energy. The watermelon juice is my favourite summer juice – unbelievably hydrating and perfect on a hot day. The pineapple juice is a great juice if you're new to juicing and want to try something semi-green! It has lots of cucumber in it, so it's full of goodness, but it also has pineapple to sweeten it up.

makes 1 glass

GLOWING GREEN JUICE

2 apples
1 cucumber
4 stalks of celery
1 fennel bulb
½ broccoli head
2-3cm piece of fresh ginger

Simply put all the ingredients through your juicer and then enjoy!

WATERMELON, CUCUMBER AND MINT JUICE

1 big wedge of watermelon (600g including the skin)
1 cucumber
small handful of fresh mint

Slice the watermelon flesh from the skin, then put it through your juicer with the cucumber and mint.

Sometimes the watermelon pips get into the juice, so you may want to quickly strain it before drinking.

PINEAPPLE, CUCUMBER AND GINGER JUICE

1 large cucumber
5cm slice of pineapple (300g)
2-3cm piece of fresh ginger

Simply put everything through the juicer and then enjoy the juice!

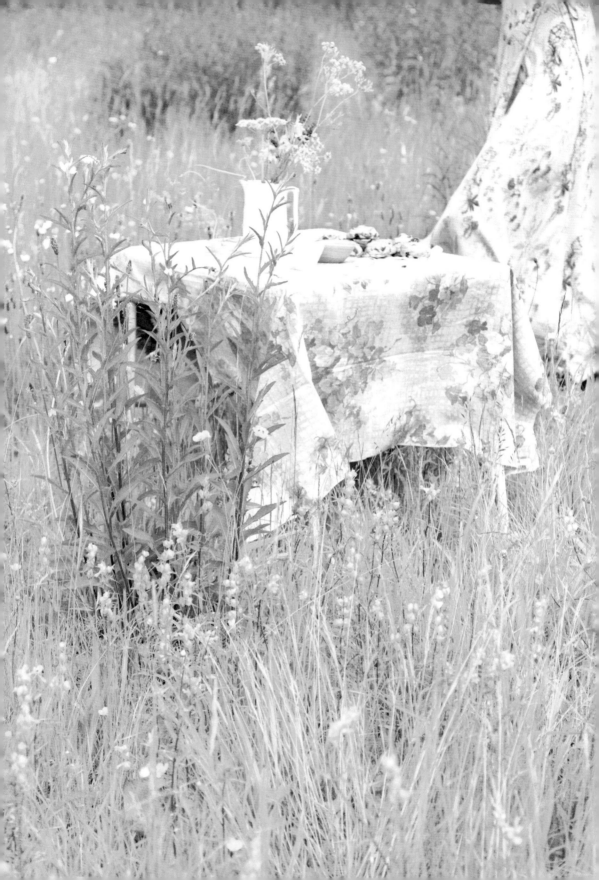

LIVING THE DELICIOUSLY ELLA WAY

putting it into practice

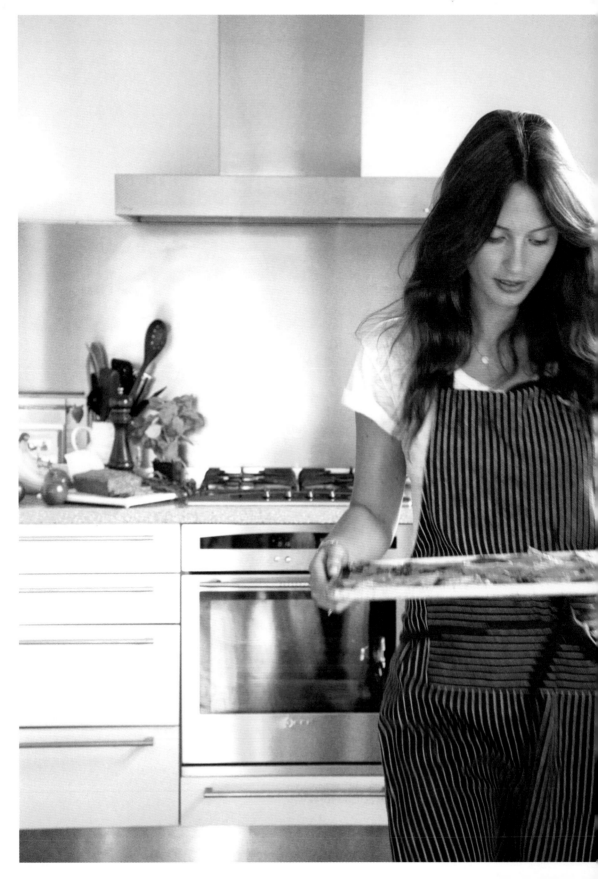

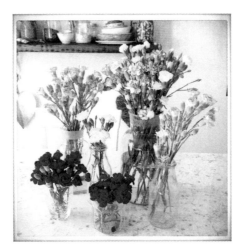

living the
Deliciously Ella way

I hope that the recipes in this book have given you some great ideas and inspiration for enjoying a delicious, yet amazingly healthy, way of life. The last thing I want to show you is how to put it all together, because I know that if you're new to a plant-based life, then the idea of throwing a dinner party, a brunch or even a girls' supper is quite daunting when you still haven't quite figured out what goes with what yet. This was a big issue for me when I first started and I did serve a few pretty random meals. It was all delicious, but not super coherent!

I hope these meal ideas will also help you with the other challenge that comes with changing your diet – convincing your friends and family to try new foods too. We all know that vegetarian food is delicious, but lots of people imagine it to be really boring, so they're not always totally open-minded about trying it. This was a huge issue for me to start with, so I do totally understand your frustration, and I found that the best way to get over this hurdle is to cook for everyone, because as soon as they try their first bite of sweet potato brownies, Thai coconut curry or guacamole, all

their preconceived ideas about veggie meals being bland will disappear and they always love the rest of the meal. I've had this experience with so many people now and it's amazing to watch. My favourite people to try this on are always my dad's friends, who are so sceptical that they actually eat a proper dinner beforehand because they're so sure that they'll hate it, but then they love it, go back for seconds or thirds, and can't stop asking questions about every ingredient – it's incredible! That's not to say that they're convinced to become gluten-free vegans overnight – they're really not – but that's not what we're aiming for either. The hope is just to spread a love of veggies and plants so that everyone starts to eat a little more of them and you can start to enjoy all these recipes with the people that you love.

The most amazing thing is that now my family and friends all adore this food too. None of them had ever eaten like this before, and it took a good few months to really introduce them to it, but now they eat it most of the time, with or without me. My parents, boyfriend and flatmates all make smoothies for breakfast almost every day; it's truly incredible to see. I've never told them that they should do this or said anything negative about what they used to eat, but they all just realised that this food tastes incredible and they feel so much better for it. They all eat meat, dairy and sugar too, which is totally fine as most of their meals are made up of Deliciously Ella goodness, so they have a great balance and I get to enjoy my food with them knowing that they love it, which makes me unbelievably happy.

Eating a plant-based diet isn't meant to socially isolate you and make you feel weird and different – these recipes are friend and family friendly! My advice would be to start introducing your friends and family to this food slowly. Try inviting them round for a meal that focuses on a dish that they're used to so it won't look so different, but we know that it has a healthy twist. Dishes like my Coconut Thai Curry (page 120), my Black and Kidney Bean Chilli (page 114) or my Butternut Squash Risotto (page 54) are all great places to start. They're all very hearty too and full of flavour, so they'll instantly bust the myth that this way of life is all about dieting, because it's not, it's about enjoyment and feeling amazing. You can also try simply adding an extra portion of fruit or veg to every meal, so a sliced banana or some berries in your morning porridge, a side of Guacamole (page 159) or Spicy Salsa (page 135) with lunch and some Easy Roast Veggies (page 128) with dinner. Making these subtle changes means that you won't suddenly feel overwhelmed by a whole new lifestyle, but you'll start getting used to eating this way and you'll feel great for the extra goodness.

The great thing is that the more you make these recipes, the more your own confidence will grow and you'll start to work out your own amazing flavour combinations and favourite meals. Once you do this, then you'll be able to create things that you know everyone else will love and will be begging to come round to dinner with you! While you get started though, I've shared all my favourite meal combinations with you, so that you can start creating amazing meals that convince everyone you know to start loving plants!

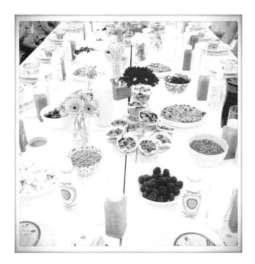

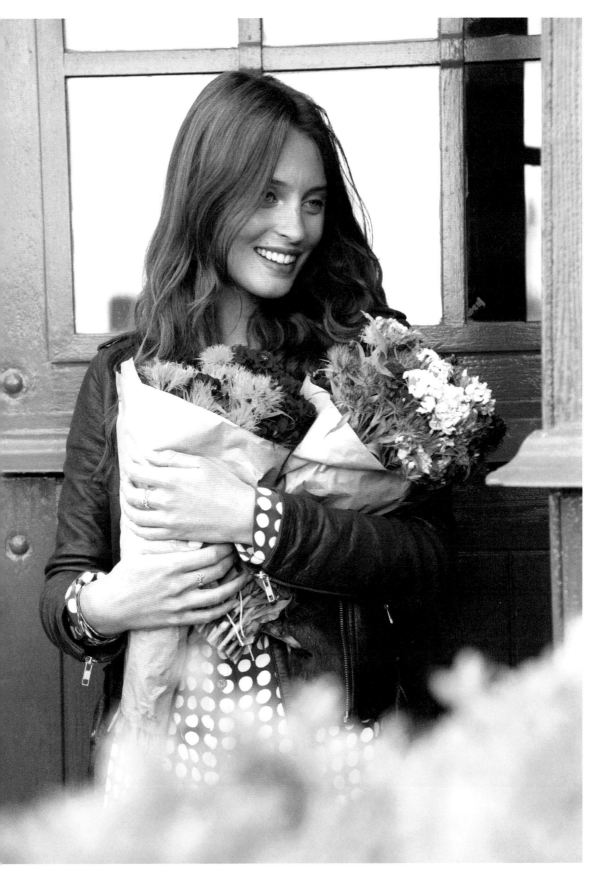

BRUNCH

I know the idea of a gluten-free, vegan brunch might sound a little dull, and in the past I would have been the first person to agree with you there, but actually you can make something totally divine that will really surprise everyone! I mean, how delicious does this sound – giant hash browns with home-made baked beans; mashed avocado with a drizzling of lime and a sprinkling of chilli flakes; fluffy sweet potato pancakes or banana waffles covered in fresh berries and maple syrup; some cinnamon-infused apple purée to eat with everything and a side of fresh fruit. There's really nothing boring about that at all! Of course, you can throw in some non-Deliciously Ella things too so that all your guests are happy. Scrambled eggs and sausages go well with everything that I've laid out, so don't worry that it's a negative thing to include them, just enjoy them alongside all the plant-based goodness.

What you'll need:
Baked Beans (page 112)
Giant Hash Brown (page 130)
Sweet Potato Pancakes (page 163) or Waffles (page 183) with berries
   and maple syrup
Apple Purée (page 19)
Avocados to mash with lime juice and chilli flakes
Fresh fruit (I normally have a big bowl of berries)
Carrot, Apple and Ginger Juice (page 220)

These recipes together create something so magical! I normally serve the savoury part of the brunch first, so the baked beans with the mashed avocado and my giant hash brown, which is cut into slices so that everyone can have some. I use the hash brown slices like toast here, spreading the avocado onto the slice and then scooping some baked beans on top. I'm quite a fan of adding a little apple purée to the savoury part too as it sweetens it up and is so delicious. I then move on to the sweet section of the meal, serving the pancakes or waffles with the fresh berries, a layer of apple purée and then a drizzling of maple syrup on the top, which is beyond incredible! Normally I'll make smoothies or juices for everyone too. My favourite brunch juice is a classic apple, carrot and ginger juice as it goes with everything.

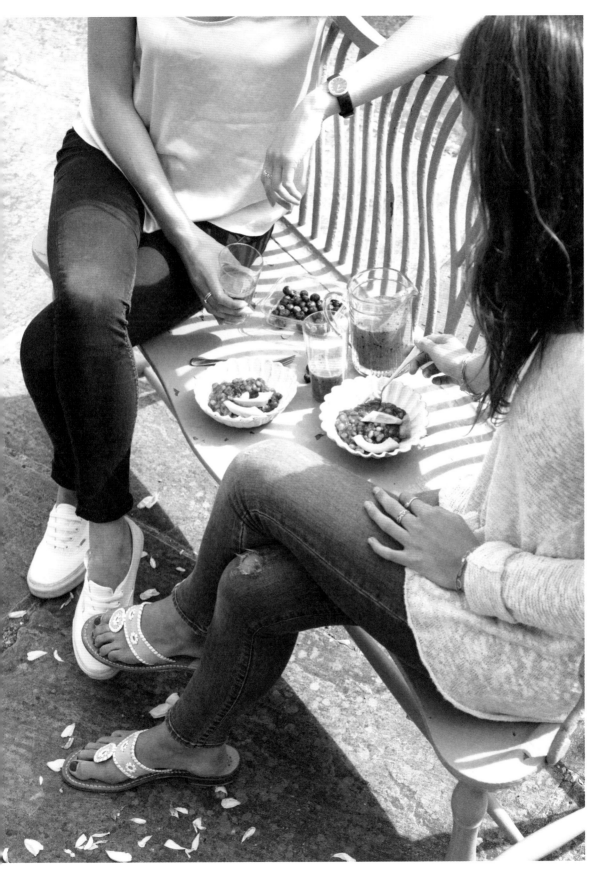

THE PERFECT DINNER PARTY: MENU ONE

My favourite dinner party meal is such a hit, even with the sceptics! I love serving a bowl of my roasted red pepper and paprika hummus with superfood crackers as nibbles, followed by a beetroot carpaccio with rocket to start. Then my Thai curry with tamari-infused brown rice and cinnamon sweet potato wedges, and for dessert, my key lime pie.

What you'll need:
Roasted Red Pepper and Paprika Hummus (page 102)
Superfood Crackers (page 82)
Beetroot Carpaccio with rocket (page 140)
Coconut Thai Curry with Chickpeas (page 120)
Sweet Potato Wedges (page 132)
Key Lime Pie (page 196)

I was absolutely terrified before the first plant-based dinner party I did. I was so sure that everyone was going to hate the food and think I was a lunatic! Luckily, it was such a success. Every last morsel of food was eaten and everyone loved all the dishes, which really gave me more confidence to keep going with this knowing that I wasn't totally mad!

With this menu there are a few things you can do to make the cooking a little easier for yourself. I roast the beetroot for the carpaccio, make the key lime pie, the hummus and bake the crackers the day before, as they don't need to be totally fresh, and then the sweet potato wedges, curry and hummus only take about an hour to go from fridge to plate, so it's pretty easy. I cut the sweet potato wedges first and put them in the oven to cook. Once they're going, I prepare the curry and start cooking that. Doing it in this order means they normally all finish cooking at the same time so they're all nice and hot and while they cook, you can make the carpaccio.

I love watching everyone eat this. It's so fun to see how much everyone loves it, especially when they're not expecting to! The key lime pie is especially fun for this as the colour is so different to a normal dessert, which always intrigues everyone. I normally withhold the ingredient list and make everyone try it first, see how much they enjoy it, and then reveal that it's actually made of avocados and they're always shocked! I tend not to tell them first so they don't make judgements without trying it. Sharing food with friends and family is just the best and it's so nice to sit around the kitchen table chatting about life while eating something delicious.

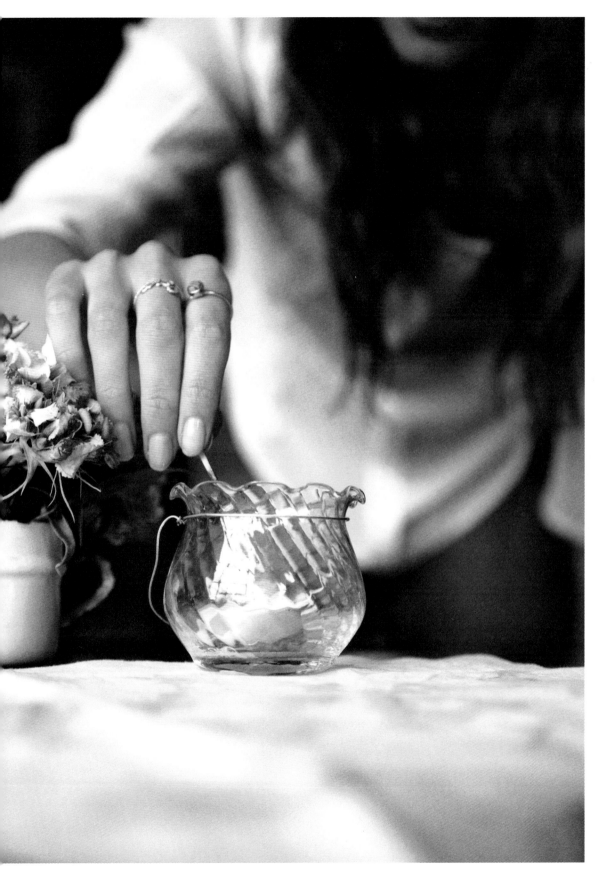

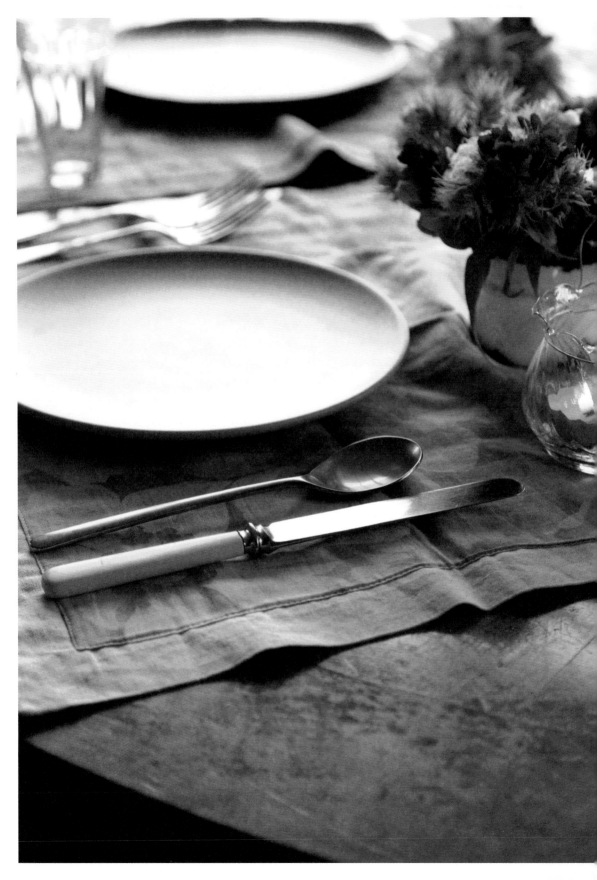

THE PERFECT DINNER PARTY: MENU TWO

If you're after a second menu because your guests loved the first so much that they want to come back for more, then this is what I'd recommend! I'd serve my amazing carrot, cashew and orange salad as a starter, followed by my roasted butternut squash risotto with a side of tahini broccoli, and then my beetroot chocolate cake with creamy coconut icing and some banana ice cream to finish.

What you'll need:

Carrot, Orange and Cashew Salad (page 139)
Butternut Squash Risotto (page 54)
Broccoli with a Tahini Dressing (page 159)
Beetroot Chocolate Cake with Coconut Frosting (page 164)
Banana Ice Cream (page 198)

This menu plan is a little quicker to prepare then the first dinner party plan, so if you're short on time, then I'd really recommend trying this one first. Both are equally delicious, so you don't need to worry about that!

One of the nice things about this meal is that the starter is really light, so you'll have extra space for the dessert, which is my favourite recipe in the whole book. It's a fun dessert to make for people that are new to plant-based eating too as it's made from beetroots, and I love being able to surprise people when they ask what's in a dish and then watch their looks of surprise when you tell them! People just never expect sweet, delicious cakes to be made of veggies and it's pretty cool to show them that you can make the most beautiful meals using only natural ingredients.

To make this dinner I start by making the carrot, cashew and orange salad as this only takes 10 to 15 minutes and it's served cold so you don't need to worry about it once it's made. Then once that's all done, I put the risotto on to cook, then while that cooks, I prepare the cake and put that in the oven too while I whizz up the icing and the ice cream and steam the broccoli. Doing it this way means that you can chat to your guests when they arrive as everything is already cooking, which should make getting dinner together a totally stress-free experience!

GIRLS' DINNER

If I'm having my girlfriends over for a casual kitchen supper, then I normally do something a bit simpler than my dinner party meal plans as I don't want to spend lots of time in the kitchen. One of my favourite meals to make is my brazil nut and rocket pesto pasta, which is peas, courgette slices and broccoli. I then make a broccoli and avocado salad on the side and finish everything off with individual mango and cashew mousses as dessert. I'm not a huge drinker so I normally serve this with fresh juice instead of wine. My pineapple, cucumber and ginger juice is especially nice with this meal as it's wonderfully light and refreshing and gives everyone a little boost of green goodness.

What you'll need:
Brazil Nut and Rocket Pesto Pasta (page 86)
Broccoli and Avocado Salad (page 148)
Simple Mango and Cashew Mousse (page 184)
Pineapple, Cucumber and Ginger Juice (page 223)

I love this menu as it's totally fuss-free and so quick to put together – everything goes from fridge to plate in less than 30 minutes. All the ingredients are available in any supermarket too; you don't need anything specific to a health-food shop or that you have to think of in advance. It's also a really easy meal to cook, as pretty much all you have to do is blend pesto, steam broccoli and blend mangoes, which I love as it means you have way more time to chat with the girls when they arrive! It also all comes out looking incredibly delicious and impressive, so you'll look like a domestic goddess!

This meal is the perfect balance between healthy and comforting. It's full of greens from the rocket, peas, courgettes and broccoli in the pasta to the avocado and broccoli in the salad and the cucumber in the juice, so everyone always leaves the meal feeling great. I also love knowing that I've just given everyone an incredible dose of vitamins and minerals! The amazing thing is that all the greens are served in ways that make them seem like 'normal' food and no one notices how healthy each dish is, as nothing about it looks intimidatingly healthy. Instead it all feels warming and comforting in a way that everyone loves and feels comfortable with. So this kind of meal is great for introducing friends to healthy food and I'm sure that all your friends will love everything you make so much that they'll soon be wanting to come back for more!

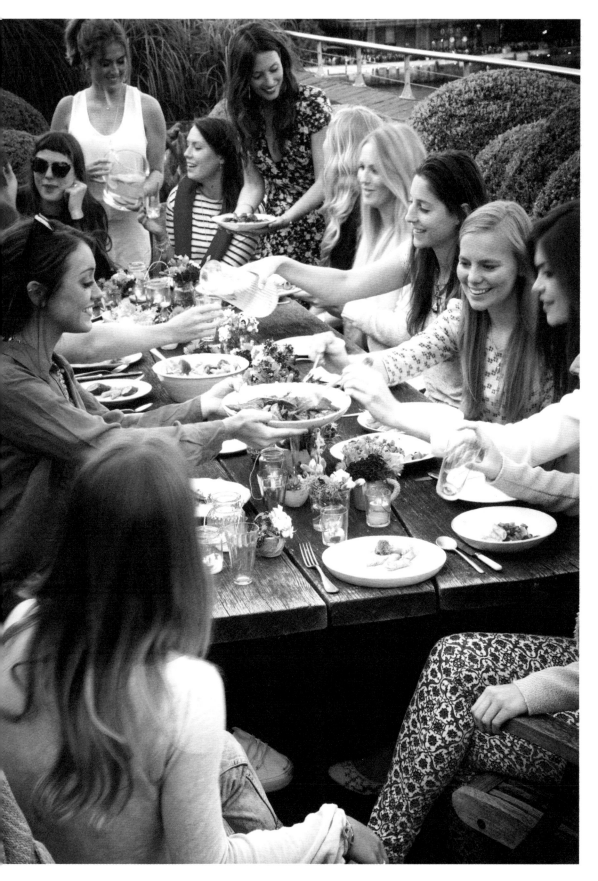

PICNICS AND HEALTHY FOOD ON THE GO

There are lots of awesome picnic ideas for summer lunches floating through the book and you can make the most beautiful spread using a mixture of them. I love having some avocado and cucumber rolls, a marinated kale salad with pomegranates, some quinoa tabbouleh, and then a couple of pots of chunky guacamole and roasted red pepper hummus, plus some crudités to dip into them. For dessert, I normally pick really easy, portable things such as blueberry muffins and almond and chia energy balls, so that there's something fruity and something chocolatey, which normally means that everyone is happy!

In terms of drinks, I love bringing big jugs of juice, normally something refreshing like my cucumber, pear and mint juice or my carrot, apple and ginger juice. I find that juice travels better than smoothies and I prefer having something lighter with my picnics as it leaves room for all the delicious food. My top tip though is to put lots of ice in the juice once it's made so that it stays fresh and cold while it travels, as warm juice isn't as delicious!

What you'll need:

Cucumber and Avocado
   Rolls (page 136)
Marinated Kale Salad
   (page 153)
Quinoa Tabbouleh
   (page 46)
Classic Guacamole
   (page 132)
Roasted Red Pepper and
   Paprika Hummus
   (page 102) with crudités
Blueberry Muffins
   (page 184)
Almond and Chia Energy
   Bites (page 72)
Cucumber, Pear and
   Mint Juice (page 220)
   or my Carrot, Apple
   and Ginger Juice (page
   220)

There's something really fun about picnic food. It's such a wonderful way to share food with friends and it's always a great way to taste a little bit of everything, which I particularly love. This is a fun way to introduce your friends and family to healthy food too, as they can sample a little of every dish and there are so many options that it doesn't matter if they don't love one of them.

All of the foods that I've suggested are really easy to transport. I simply put them in individual Tupperware boxes and then they stay fresh until you're ready to eat them. It's all food that tastes just as delicious hours after you've made it, so it doesn't need to be eaten straight away.

This also means that all the dishes I've suggested for a picnic will work perfectly for work lunches too, if you're looking to take food on the go with you. I normally make a big batch of them all on a Sunday and then store them in my fridge so that each morning I can scoop up a few spoonfuls of each, put them in a Tupperware box and then enjoy them for lunch later on. It means that lunch will always be a delicious meal and you won't feel deprived or hungry, as you'll be prepared with great food. This is so important if you're trying to eat well and want to avoid the sugary snacks in the office, because if you're not happy and satisfied with your food then it's almost impossible to resist the sugar!

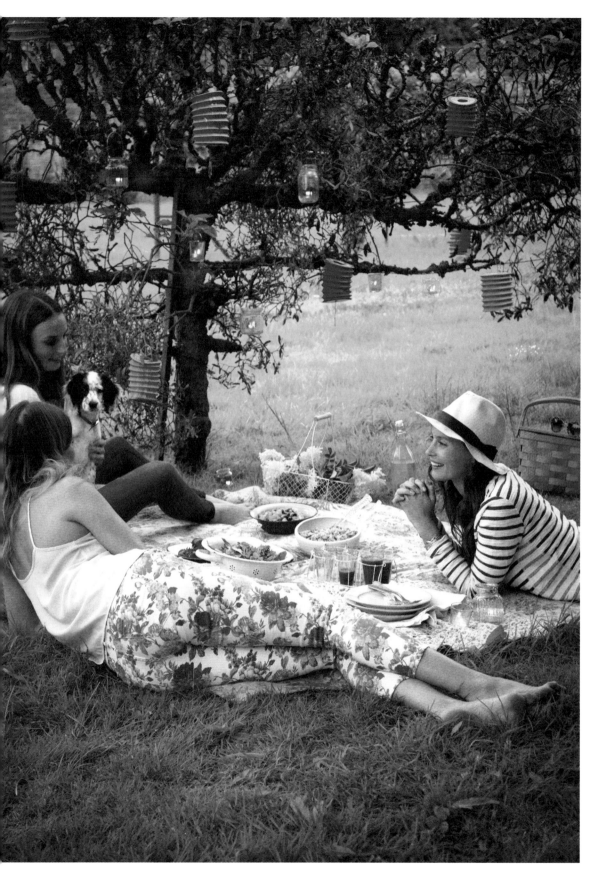

SUNDAY ROAST

The final meal that I'd love to give you some ideas for is a Sunday roast, as I know that it is such a popular weekend tradition. I love to serve my roast potatoes with rosemary and thyme; my easy roasted veggies, my stuffed chestnut mushrooms with pine nuts and sun-dried tomatoes and my marinated kale salad on the side, for some green goodness.

Then, of course, you have to have a crumble for dessert, so I make my apple and blackberry crumble with one-ingredient banana ice cream on the side – it's amazing!

What you'll need:

Perfect Roast Potatoes (page 132)

Easy Roast Veggies (page 128)

Stuffed Chestnut Mushrooms (page 150)

Marinated Kale Salad (page 153)

Apple and Blackberry Crumble (page 189)

Banana Ice Cream (page 198)

I know that a vegetarian Sunday roast is a little unconventional, but I promise you that it really does taste better than anything else! Every dish is delicious and so rich in flavour that you'll be very happy, plus together they're really filling, so I don't think you'll feel that you're missing much by skipping the meat.

If you or other members of your family aren't ready to move away from meat just yet, then you can always make a compromise and cook some meat alongside all these sides in order to ensure that everyone's happy. That's what I do with my family and it works really well. My mum's a veggie so she eats exactly the same as me, but the others love their meat from time to time, so we cook Deliciously Ella sides with a roast chicken or fillet of beef. Everyone gobbles up plant-based goodness and our plates all look pretty similar, so I don't feel weird or isolated for eating this way, which is really important if it's going to become a way of life for you. This meal is so good that we've made it for lunch on Christmas Day for the last couple of years and it's always a huge hit with all our friends and extended family, so I'm sure that all of your family will love it too!

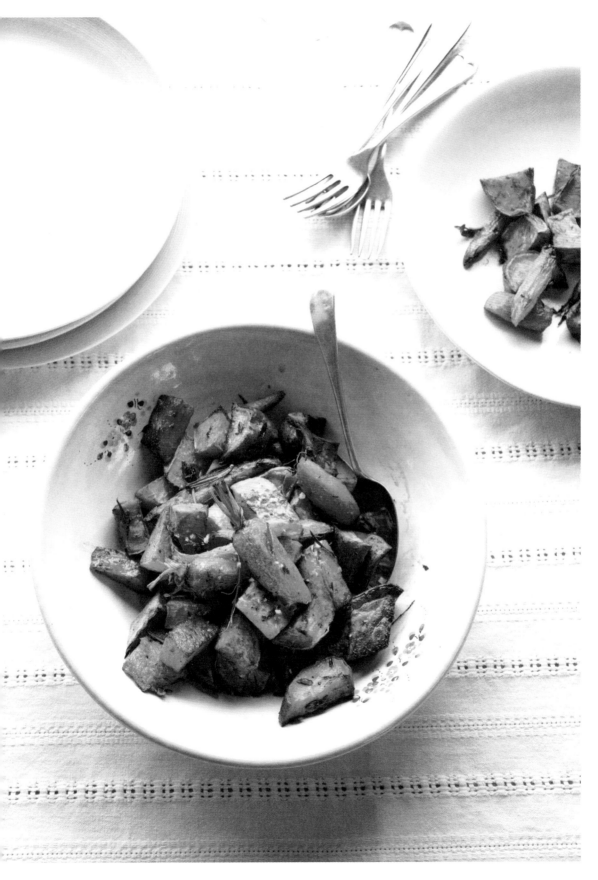

MY FAVOURITE RESOURCES

SHOPS IN LONDON

Planet Organic – this is a health nut's dream, it's full of the most amazing products and you'll want to buy everything in there! They sell absolutely everything you need to make all my recipes, plus lots of amazing snacks from raw chocolate to kale chips and freshly made smoothies and juices. They have several sites around London, my favourite one is on Westbourne Grove, but there are also amazing stores on Torrington Place, in Wandsworth, in Islington and Devonshire Square.

Whole Foods – this is another amazing health-food shop, it's a lot bigger than Planet Organic so it's harder to navigate but they also sell absolutely everything you could ever need in their shops in Kensington, Piccadilly and Fulham.

Revital on Wigmore Street – this is my favourite little health-food shop, it's pretty small but unbelievably well stocked so it's really easy to find everything you need. They also sell everything you need for any of these recipes.

Holland and Barrett – a great place to go for nuts, nut butters, coconut oil and maple syrup. They're all over the country so it's normally easy to find one near you. Don't buy your dates from there though, as they're coated in vegetable oil and very hard, so won't work in these recipes.

Borough Market – this is the most beautiful market in the world and it sells the most delicious fresh fruit and veggies, so worth visiting to stock up on groceries plus amazing olive oil, tapenades, hummus and fresh pestos.

ONLINE SHOPS

Goodnessdirect.com – they sell absolutely everything and it's delivered straight to your door, which is great for staying organised so that you always have everything you need to eat deliciously healthy food.

Planetorganic.com – an online version of their shop, so it's a great place to stock up on goodness.

Amazon – I know it's a sell out but Amazon are pretty amazing for buying your supplies in bulk at great prices. You can buy a kilo of organic almonds, for example, for £14, or three huge jars of tahini for £10. I do big orders from them every few months so that I'm always stocked up on my pantry essentials.

FAVOURITE WEBSITES

These are three of the most beautiful, inspiring blogs you'll ever see!

Greenkitchenstories.com

Mynewroots.org

Sproutedkitchen.com

My other favourite website is Mind Body Green, it's a collection of articles which all focus on health, food and wellbeing – it's very inspiring and full of amazing information.

Mindbodygreen.com

FAVOURITE BOOKS

Crazy Sexy Diet by Kris Carr – the first book I ever read on this topic, and the most inspirational. Kris shares her story of how she healed her inoperable cancer through diet – just amazing and a very easy, very positive read.

Clean by Dr. Alejandro Junger – a fascinating book written by a doctor disillusioned by modern medicine, all about how we should treat our bodies with a clean diet and lifestyle for optimum health. Also easy to read and really interesting.

The China Study by Dr. T. Colin Campbell – a lot of science in this book so less easy to read, more something to dip in and out of but a serious must read. It details the largest study on nutrition ever conducted and the results of it. It really changed my outlook on food and helped me understand why I needed to eat the way I do.

The Blood Sugar Solution by Dr. Mark Hyman – less 'extreme' then the others and offers a very understandable, very straightforward insight into how to clean up your diet. If you're very new to healthy eating this is very helpful.

Ultra-Metabolism by Dr. Mark Hyman – similar to *The Blood Sugar Solution* and great for all the same reasons, but gives a new insight into how our metabolism works and a big stress on how all calories are not equal!

The Beauty Detox Solution by Kimberly Snyder – lovely, very easy book to read that explains how energy needs to be freed from our digestive systems to give us optimum health and therefore optimum beauty. Explains how a plant-based diet will do this.

Mind Over Medicine by Lissa Rankin – this is amazing, it's all about how powerful the mind is and how important its role is in healing. If you're struggling with illness then I couldn't recommend this more, it really helped me.

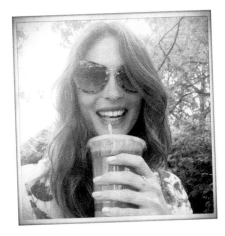

PLACES TO EAT AND DRINK IN LONDON

Mildreds, Lexington Street, Soho

Manna, Primrose Hill

Retreat Café, Fulham

Tri-yoga café, Kings Road

Vantra, Tottenham Court Road

The Good Life Eatery, Sloane Avenue

Borough Market, London Bridge

Juice Tonic bar, Piccadily

The Wild Food Café, Covent Garden

Roots and Bulbs, Marylebone High Street

Tibits, Heddon Street

Duke of York market, The Kings Road– rainforest creations, raw snacks and coconut water

Laborganic, Covent Garden

Whole Foods

Planet Organic

MY KITCHEN EQUIPMENT

Magimix Food Processor – these are the best food processors ever, it's a life long investment and so worth it, you can make literally anything in them!

Vitamix Blender – I use a Vitamix Blender, they are pretty expensive but if you're going to use it everyday then it's worth the investment as they are amazing!

Philips Blender – If you're looking for a less expensive blender Philips make really good ones for about £80 which will do everything that you need. It may seem like a lot but the blenders that cost less aren't that strong and so they struggle to break everything down into a smooth, creamy mix.

Magimix and Sage Juicers – both Magimix and Sage make great juicers, which are very easy to wash up!

Spiralz Vegetable Spiralizer – this is the spiralizer I use, you can buy it on Amazon and it's amazing, courgette noodles are life changing!

FREQUENTLY ASKED QUESTIONS

These are the questions I get asked every day, so I thought it would be helpful to share my responses here. I hope they give you a little more insight into my lifestyle and some inspiration to live this way!

HOW DO I GET STARTED?

I think it's all about starting slowly, so that the diet gradually becomes a natural part of your routine and eventually a way of life. Just making one small change a day is amazing, such as adding in one new serving of fruit or veg a day – some sweet potato wedges or guacamole make an insanely delicious addition to any meal and they're such an easy place to start. Whizzing up a smoothie in the morning is incredible too as it always starts you off on the right track for a positive day, while giving you an abundance of goodness and energy. Making small changes every week over a few months will result in huge changes but you won't feel overwhelmed by them!

WHAT SHOULD I EAT LESS OF?

As humans we're all different, we want and need different things and listening to your own body is the best thing that you can do. There are some things, however, that aren't great for any of us and it's those things that we should try and eat less of – mainly refined sugar, processed foods, additives and preservatives, gluten and dairy. Saying goodbye to these things will really help you look and feel your absolute best, and I promise the food really does still taste good! When it comes to fish, eggs and meat I believe that we should eat less of them as they're much harder on our bodies both because they're more acidic and because they're much more difficult to digest – that being said, you have to do what's right for you. I feel a million times better without them, but if you want to include them in your diet then please do – just focus on where they came from, and try to have one meal a day that's plant-based.

DO I HAVE TO FOLLOW A STRICT PLANT-BASED DIET TO GET THE BENEFITS?

Absolutely not, any changes no matter how small will have awesome benefits – you really don't have to go the whole way, just make it work for you. My advice would be to try and eat this way at least half the time, do it for the meals that you eat at home or work – so your weekday breakfasts, work lunches and any meals that you eat alone. Then when you go out to dinner with friends enjoy the food, order the best pizza or chocolate cake and truly savour all the delicious flavours. We've gotten so used to eating bad versions of these foods all the time, instead I think we should start eating to nourish our bodies most of the time so that we feel amazing and then really enjoy the other food for its flavours, not for its convenience. Please don't feel guilty when you go out and enjoy the food either, this way of eating really isn't a diet, so it's not an all or nothing situation – it's simply just about loving your body and if that includes chocolate cake and pizza once a week, then that's great!

DO YOU EAT THIS WAY ALL THE TIME?

I do eat this way all the time, but for me this way of eating has been my way of healing and putting my illness into remission so I'm conscious of keeping it this way. This doesn't mean that you have to eat this way all the time though and I'm absolutely not judging you if you don't – we all have to do what's right for us individually to stay happy and healthy.

DO YOU COUNT CALORIES?

Never, ever! I believe in counting goodness, not calories. If you eat amazing natural food then you really don't need to think about calories, they become irrelevant. Instead think about the range of vitamins and minerals that you're eating. Besides, not all calories are created equal, an avocado is in no shape or form equal to a chocolate bar even if they can have similar calorie contents. An avocado contains wonderful compounds that will nourish your body, give you glowing skin, and make you feel happy. It's also much easier to digest so it will give you amazing energy too.

HOW CAN I EAT THIS WAY ON A BUDGET?

There's an assumption that healthy eating has to be really expensive, but I promise you it really doesn't. I actually spend less now than I did before. The things I eat on a day-to-day basis are really inexpensive; I focus on seasonal veggies, grains and beans – all of which are very cheap. Mixing brown rice, for example, with black beans, a little tamari and tomato puree and then serving the rice with avocado costs almost nothing, tastes amazing and fills you with goodness. The main thing is not to fall for all the gluten-free products in supermarkets, as these are unbelievably expensive and full of rubbish too! Eating seasonally is important too as mangoes and pineapples will always cost more than carrots or beetroots during the winter, likewise only buy fresh berries in the summer as they'll cost you a fortune out of season and taste of very little – buy frozen ones instead in the winter. The one thing that is more expensive is baking, there's no way round this really as we're using whole, nutritious ingredients which just do cost more – but if you're only baking once a week this all evens out. Besides, you save a lot of money not buying chocolate bars, snacks and crisps when you're out and about too.

HOW DO I MANAGE EATING ON THE GO?

My answer to this is really boring, but staying healthy when you're out and about and really busy is all about organisation. I take a couple of hours every Sunday to prepare a few different dishes, which will power me through the week. My staples are a big batch of grains (either brown rice, quinoa or buckwheat), some cinnamon and paprika sweet potato wedges, some lentils, lots of homemade hummus and my marinated kale salad. I'll then buy some fresh ingredients, normally avocados, cucumbers, rocket, olives and tomatoes and then each morning I'll fill a Tupperware with a mixture of all of these things – the whole thing takes just five minutes and makes lunch time so much more fun, plus it gives you all the energy you need to beat the all-too-common afternoon slump. It's much cheaper than buying lunch out too! For snacks I normally focus on my energy balls, my crackers, and hummus with crudités or rice cakes – again these won't take you long to make but they'll help you feel amazing all day, every day.

WHAT IF I'M REALLY BUSY AND DON'T HAVE THE TIME TO COOK ALL THIS FOOD?

It's important to make the time, I totally understand being incredibly busy makes it seem like being healthy is impossible but we can all sacrifice something to find two hours one day a week to prepare everything you need to stay healthy all week. If you do this then for the rest of the week you only need five to ten minutes to make something awesome. Trust me, it's so worth sacrificing one thing to do this – it makes such a huge difference!

WHAT DO YOU DO WHEN YOU'RE OUT WITH FRIENDS; DO YOU GET FRUSTRATED EATING OUT?

I found eating out with friends really difficult to start with – for me it was probably the biggest obstacle I faced when I changed my diet. It's hard feeling different to everyone else, and even harder not to worry that people are judging you. It took me about six months to adjust to being different, accept it and then finally embrace it. Once you understand why you're doing this it's easier to explain it to other people too. It's also important to stress to whoever you're with that you're absolutely not judging them – you're doing this simply because it makes you feel amazing, which makes you a happier and nicer person to be around. One of the first things I did to ease the awkwardness of being different was to invite my friends over to try all the food I was experimenting with, so that they could see how delicious it was. They all absolutely loved it and have really embraced it, lots of them now incorporate aspects of this diet in their life too which makes it much easier. When I eat out I'll call the restaurant first and just let them know so that I don't have to make a fuss when I arrive and then I just order all the sides on the menu, which normally means I get a lovely plate of roasted potatoes, roasted veggies and sautéed spinach – all of which tastes delicious. You have to accept that it won't be the most exciting meal of your life, but it means you still get a plate of food and you can enjoy being out with friends!

DO YOU EVER 'CHEAT' AND EAT 'BAD' FOOD?

This is a question I get asked all the time, and the answer is no – not because I'm really boring, but because I don't want to. This isn't a diet for me; it's a lifestyle, which I absolutely adore. I do get sweet cravings, but they're for sweet potato brownies or dates with almond butter, rather than Haribo. It takes a few months for your taste buds to adjust and for this way of eating to become a totally natural part of your life, but once it does you just won't think of 'cheat' foods, they'll start to seem kind of gross actually, and you'll feel so truly amazing that they'll have no appeal at all.

WHAT SUGAR SUBSTITUTES DO YOU USE?

Sugar is such a complicated topic and there really are a hundred different arguments for and against almost anything sugary. Everyone agrees that refined sugar is bad, it's inflammatory and does crazy things to your blood sugar levels, but not everyone agrees on everything else so you have to find what works for you! I use either pure maple syrup, raw honey or date syrup in all my recipes and as toppings for things like pancakes and porridge. All three are totally natural, contain vitamins and minerals and don't do crazy things to your blood sugar in the way that white sugar does. I don't use them every day though, maybe twice a week or so but my taste buds don't crave sugary things as much now – when I first started doing this I used one of the three at least once a day while I got used to not eating refined sugar.

SHOULD I LIMIT MY FRUIT INTAKE?

I don't put any restrictions on what I eat, I'll eat any fruit, vegetable, grain, seed, nut, bean etc at any time in whatever quantity I'm craving. I found that putting rules into this lifestyle made it too restrictive and I didn't enjoy it. Fruit does contain sugar, but it's natural, it doesn't do crazy things to your blood sugar and it contains unbelievable amounts of goodness, which our bodies need. I thrive on fruit and absolutely love it: it's nature's candy! Some people find too much fruit gives them upset stomachs, so listen to your body – if it makes you feel good then embrace it, if too much doesn't feel amazing then just enjoy a piece or two.

WHAT DO YOU DO WHEN YOU TRAVEL?

I always travel with a small travel blender when I'm away for a few days, I know that's quite sad but it makes a huge difference. Once I arrive at my destination I'll buy a selection of fruit, vegetables and nuts which I can then blend every morning so that even if it's hard to get good food the rest of the day I know I've had three or four portions of goodness already, which keeps me feeling awesome. I also travel with some bread, normally a brown rice and sunflower seed bread from a company called Biona, so that I can always eat a few slices of that with mashed avocado or banana in case I can't find anything else to eat. The final thing I do is bring a selection of snacks – granola bars, date and nut bars, nuts and crackers – so that I'm never hungry!

WHAT DOES A DAY ON YOUR PLATE LOOK LIKE?

Each day is different and I try to mix up my meals so that I get a great variety of vitamins and minerals. I start every morning with a smoothie though, lunch is normally a mix of whatever I've prepared for the week, which takes just five minutes to put together as it's all already prepared – maybe some brown rice with marinated kale, mashed avocado, lentils and sweet potato. Dinner is when I get more creative and spend more time in the kitchen; I'll often make a curry, a risotto or a stir-fry, as I love having something hearty and warming after a busy day. My snacks throughout the day are pretty simple: if I'm out and about I'll often buy a fresh juice or carry some trail mix or a couple of energy balls with me, if I'm at home I often snack on homemade hummus with crudités or rice cakes.

HOW CAN I EAT ENOUGH PROTEIN ON A PLANT-BASED DIET?

If you don't eat animal products then you need to be conscious of your protein intake. Saying that, it's unbelievably easy to eat more than enough protein as there's protein in so many different foods. I eat at least one protein source with every meal, as this keeps my blood sugar levels steady and my energy levels wonderfully high! The best plant-based protein sources are: all forms of pulses (beans, chickpeas and hummus, lentils), quinoa, dark green leafy veggies (like kale and spinach), nuts and seeds, hemp (powder or seeds) and spirulina. Most vegetables have protein too: an avocado, for example, has about ten grams of protein in it, while a cup of broccoli has five

grams and a cup of peas has about ten grams. So it's easy to eat lots of protein, you just need to be mindful that you're including a variety of these foods in your diet. I normally have almond butter, spirulina and hemp powder in my morning smoothie, my snacks always include nuts and seeds of some kind, and my lunches and dinners include a mixture of all the other sources.

WHAT ARE THE BEST PLANT-BASED SOURCES OF CALCIUM?

Lots of people worry that giving up dairy will mean that they become calcium deficient, but it's actually so easy to eat lots of calcium and you just have to be mindful of where to get it – just like plant-based protein. Lots of studies also show that plant-based sources of calcium are actually better for us too as they're not acidic at all and so the calcium stays in our bones, rather than being leached into the blood to alkalinise the body. The best veggie sources of calcium are sesame seeds and tahini, sunflower seeds, hemp seeds (or powder), almonds and almond butter, brazil nuts, kale, rocket, broccoli, fennel, figs, oranges and beans. All these foods are delicious so it's not difficult to add them in!

WHAT ARE THE BEST PLANT-BASED SOURCES OF IRON?

Iron is a really essential nutrient that lots of people, both meat eaters and vegetarians alike, are deficient in. It's so important because it enables oxygen to be carried around the body, which gives you energy. So if you're feeling exhausted try adding more of these foods to your diet. The best plant based sources are: all pulses (lentils, chickpeas, beans), spinach, kale, Swiss chard, spirulina, quinoa, beetroot, broccoli, peas, sesame seeds and tahini, sunflower seeds, pumpkin seeds, cashews, almonds, dates and raisins. Eating your iron-rich foods with foods that contain lots of vitamin C is always a great idea too, as the vitamin C increases the body's ability to absorb the iron.

WHAT ARE YOUR THOUGHTS ON ORGANIC FOOD?

I don't think you should stress over whether your food is organic, the first thing to think about is whether it is natural and nourishing! Organic food is more expensive, so if it's out of your budget then don't worry about it – it's much better for you to eat non-organic veggies then no veggies at all. Personally I try to buy 'the dirty dozen' organic, as these are the fruits and veggies that absorb the most chemicals from the soil, so if you're going to buy anything organic then start with the things on this list – apples, strawberries, grapes, celery, peaches, spinach, peppers, nectarines, cucumbers, potatoes, tomatoes and jalapeno peppers. On the other hand 'the clean fifteen', which are the fruits and veggies that absorb the least amount of pesticides, are things that you don't have to worry so much about. These include mushrooms, sweet potatoes, melon, grapefruit, kiwi, aubergines, asparagus, mangoes, papayas, peas, cabbage, avocados, pineapples, onions and sweetcorn.

WHAT ARE YOUR THOUGHTS ON FOOD COMBINING, RAW DIETS, JUICE CLEANSES ETC?

I think there's always a danger of taking healthy eating too far, it's meant to be a fun experience not a chore. I know lots of people would think that my diet is restrictive, and to some extent it is as I don't eat lots of the food groups that make up a typical Western diet. I don't feel it's restrictive at all though, as I know that I can eat any fruit, vegetable, nut, seed or grain at any time with anything – which is really important for me, as it allows me to love the way I eat. I tried food combining and a raw diet for a few weeks each and honestly I hated both, I found them so restrictive, I didn't feel any better and I wasn't excited about my meals! Saying that we're all different, and if they make you feel great then that's awesome, but personally I'm not a huge fan of either. Likewise juice cleanses are a tricky subject, I know they're very popular at the moment, but I think they're something you have to be careful of. Juicing is amazing, it floods your body with goodness and provides you with so many amazing vitamins and minerals. But I would say have a juice a day instead of doing a three-day cleanse where you only drink juice, as you'll probably be hungry and grumpy! If you want to do a cleanse then do a day of liquids, so juices, smoothies and soups – that way you won't be hungry, so you'll stay happy all day but you'll still give yourself a crazy amount of goodness, while also allowing your digestive system to take a break and reset itself.

DO YOU TAKE ANY SUPPLEMENTS?

When I was healing I saw the most amazing naturopath at the Hale Clinic who looked at all my symptoms and did some tests to see how different areas of my body were working, she then prescribed me a three-month course of supplements to support my healing. This did absolute wonders for me and really helped the healing process. I don't take any supplements anymore though, but I do take spirulina every day which I find really boosts my energy. Supplements are a very personal thing and we all need different things to support our own bodies, so I'd really advise going to see a naturopath to guide you through this.

CAN I LOSE WEIGHT EATING THIS WAY?

Absolutely, eating a wholefood, plant-based diet is an amazing way to get to your natural weight. Taking out gluten, processed food, animal products and refined sugar allows your digestive system to work a million times better so everything will be digested faster and more effectively, which allows you to lose weight. Don't focus on counting calories or fat though, focus on eating three proper meals a day filled only with goodness and you'll see amazing results not just in the way that your clothes fit but in the way your skin looks and, most importantly, in the way you feel.

CAN I GAIN WEIGHT EATING THIS WAY?

Yes, if you want to gain weight than you can also do this in a healthy way eating a plant-based diet. Focus on eating big portions, as this kind of food is very easy to digest so you will need lots of it. I would eat lots of the following at every meal: healthy fats – avocados, coconut oil, nuts, nut butters, seeds and olive oil; lots of starchy fruits and veg – sweet potatoes, carrots, squash, beetroots, bananas, mangoes; lots of grains – brown rice, buckwheat, quinoa; and lots of beans/legumes – chickpeas, beans, lentils. If you have a good mix of them all in big quantities at least three times a day then your body can put on healthy weight. Then try to have a snack two or three times a day, things like rice cakes with nut butter and banana, energy balls, hummus and crackers or dates and dried fruit.

DO YOU DRINK ALCOHOL?

When I was very ill I totally stopped drinking and I didn't touch a drop of alcohol for about a year so I got totally used to not drinking. Then as I began to heal I started to feel so good that I didn't want to do anything to sabotage that, so I continued to stay away from it. I now drink once a month or so at occasions where I want to run around all night with friends and so it's worth feeling a little worse for wear the next day. It's awkward at first to be the non-drinker and people often respond quite weirdly to it, but if it makes you feel good then embrace it! When I drink I drink really good quality vodka on the rocks with lemon juice and ice, it's delicious and very pure. Saying that, if you love your wine then please enjoy it, don't feel guilty – maybe just drink a little less and try to have a couple of days a week without alcohol.

WHY AREN'T PEANUTS INCLUDED IN THE BOOK?

I don't eat peanuts because sadly peanuts are especially susceptible to mould and fungal invasions which can be carcinogenic as well as contributors to candida overgrowth. It's not that I think eating peanuts every now and again is bad, but I eat a lot of nuts and nut butter, and so in that quantity it's not great to be eating so many peanuts.

WHY IS THERE NO TOFU IN YOUR BOOK?

The first reason is that I simply don't love the taste of tofu, it's bland and has a strange texture which just doesn't agree with me! The other reason, though, is that whilst it does have some great health benefits these are often outweighed by the less healthy elements of it. Tofu is actually quite a processed food and it's also made from soy, which is often genetically modified – something that I don't love.

DID ANYTHING ELSE HELP YOUR HEALING?

It took me about eighteen months after changing to a totally plant-based, wholefoods diet (with no gluten, dairy, refined sugar, meat, anything processed) to feel well again, and I started really slowly – it absolutely wasn't uphill the whole way either, but it was the best thing I've ever done! I combined the diet with daily exercise (starting with just ten minutes' walking a day, building up to exercising five times a week for about an hour – yoga, pilates, a lot of walking and some gym). I also saw a naturopath who did wonders with supplements to support the areas of my body that weren't working – this was really essential to the process and something I couldn't recommend more if you're struggling with an illness. The three approaches together were magical and they put my illness totally into remission – on a day-to-day basis I have no symptoms and feel amazing, but I am careful to continue to eat well, sleep well and exercise every day to maintain this.

INDEX

First published in Great Britain in 2015
by Yellow Kite
An imprint of Hodder & Stoughton
An Hachette UK company

7

A CIP catalogue record for this title is available from the British Library
Hardback ISBN 978 1 444 79500 4
eBook ISBN 978 1 444 79502 8

Publisher: Liz Gough
Editorial Assistant: Emily Robertson
Copy Editor: Kay Halsey
Index: Isobel McLean
Design and Art Direction: Miranda Harvey
Photo Shoot Co-ordinator: Rebecca Coles
Photography: Clare Winfield
Food Stylist: Rosie Reynolds
Stylist: Polly Webb-Wilson
Make-up Artist: Laurey Simmons

With thanks to Anthropologie for the loan of some of the props

Photographs on pages 3, 5, 23, 31, 35, 67, 91, 111, 146, 157, 174, 176, 192, 195, 204, 216, 230 courtesy of Ella Woodward

Printed and bound by CPI Group (UK) Ltd, Croydon, CR0 4YY

Hodder & Stoughton Ltd
338 Euston Road
London NW1 3BH

www.hodder.co.uk

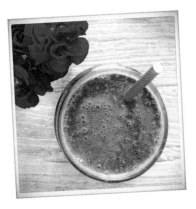

THANK YOU

My journey back to health has been such a crazy process and I could never have done it without the amazing people I have around me or my incredible blog followers, so I'd really like to take a minute to thank you all because there is no way that there would be a book without you.

First and foremost I'd like to say thank you to anyone that has read or followed Deliciously Ella. Honestly, I still can't believe how many of you have looked at my blog over the last two and a half years, it's really crazy and I'm so grateful for all your love and support, it's been so incredibly inspiring. I've read all your emails, comments, tweets, Instagram messages and Facebook posts and each one has been amazing. I love seeing the photos of all your creations and hearing how much you love the recipes. It's amazing knowing that Deliciously Ella has made a difference to your life and helped you on your own journeys to health and happiness.

Thank you to my family for being so fantastic throughout this process – you really are just the best people ever and have been so incredibly supportive of Deliciously Ella right from the beginning, even when you were the only people reading the blog!

Thank you Felix, Alex and Olivia for always being there for me. I will always be so grateful to you for your incredible love and support – you truly saved me from going crazy when I was ill and really inspired me to get well again. Thank you for seeing me through the most challenging parts of my journey and for making life so much more fun!

Thank you to my incredible friends Cressy, Oli, Chloe, Gabs, Chess, India, Lucy and Imogen for taste-testing almost every recipe in this book! Writing this wouldn't have been nearly so much fun without all your wonderful love and enthusiasm, and all our amazing Deliciously Ella dinners.

Thank you to Annie for helping me grow

Deliciously Ella and for totally saving my sanity over the last year! Working together has been so fun and I'm so grateful for all your awesome ideas.

Thank you to my wonderful agents, Cathryn and Jo, and my amazing publisher, Liz, for believing in Deliciously Ella and making this all possible. And thank you to the amazing team that put this beautiful book together – Miranda, Clare and Rosie – I'm so grateful for all the work you put into this to make it look so incredible and really bring all the recipes to life.

And finally thank you to Kris Carr, who unknowingly inspired me to change my life: thank you for sharing your story with the world and allowing thousands of people to feel amazing again.

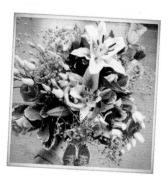

FOLLOW DELICIOUSLY ELLA

www.deliciouslyella.com

 instagram.com/DeliciouslyElla

 www.facebook.com/Deliciouslyella

 @DeliciouslyElla

 www.youtube.com – search Deliciously Ella

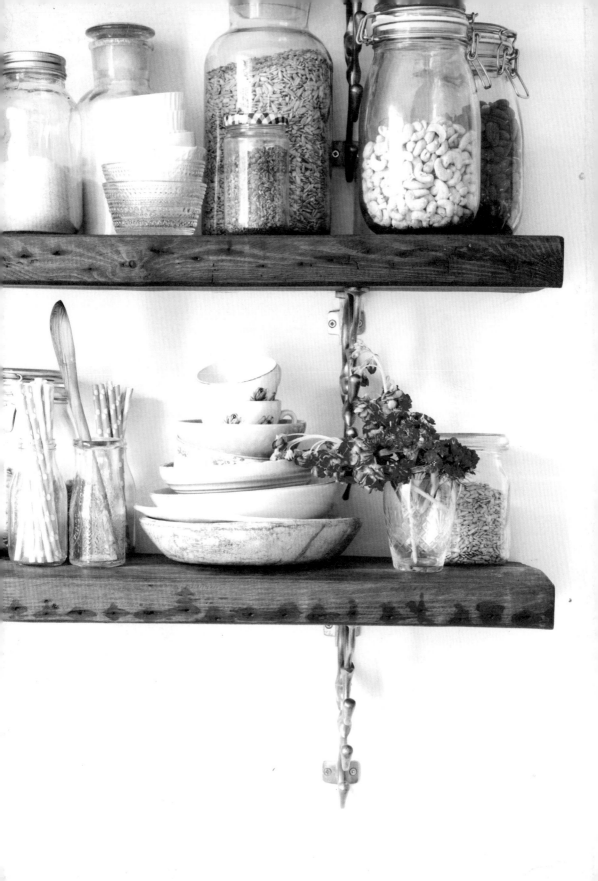